HOW TO BEAT CANCER

The agony, the ecstasy...repeat.

Victor dos Santos

ISBN-13: 9798665151571
ISBN-10: 1477123456

Cover design by: Victor dos Santos
Library of Congress Control Number: 2018675309
Printed in the United States of America

Dedicated to the special individuals that made our small miracle possible.

Cancer cannot be beaten alone.

CONTENTS

FOREWORD

*"Hope is being able to see that there is light despite
all of the darkness" – Desmond Tutu*

Sometimes it is surprisingly easy to ask: "Why me?" I often found
myself falling into this futile trap when I was diagnosed with a
rare tumour at the age of thirteen. Constant questions like this
would endlessly swirl around my head and keep me up all night
long. However, whilst desperately attempting to try find the answers, I was able to come to the realization that I was not the first
person in history to suffer from a rare disease.

Susan Sontag aptly captured the true essence of a human experience with illness. She stated that "everyone who is born holds
dual citizenship, in the kingdom of the well and in the kingdom
of the sick. Although we all prefer to use only the good passport,
sooner or later each of us is obliged, at least for a spell, to identify
ourselves as citizens of that other place". Cancer is not a novel
concept to humans and yet there is still a great deal of information that medical enquiry fails to explain. Nevertheless, being
diagnosed with cancer or a rare disease does not necessarily always equate to being handed a death sentence. Although, it is not
a pleasant experience being told that you have fallen victim to
the body's very own malady, it is a liberating task to know that
you are not alone and that there are always strategies you can
adopt to combat your disease.

My mother always quelled my anxiety by constantly reminding

me that everything that happened was part of the inexplicable "journey of life". It is increasingly difficult to know where the final destination of your own journey might end. We are not always able to choose the picture-perfect life we imagined for ourselves, albeit we can do what is best for ourselves in the present moment. Each day that unfolds will present its own new challenges, but it is of paramount importance to acknowledge that there will always be alternative options available to consider when dealing with them.

Sometimes you will feel like you are helplessly imprisoned in a room of absolute darkness, but this book will help to illuminate your struggle by providing various steps to follow if you either suspect or are diagnosed with a life-changing illness. This story is not just my own personal, coming-of-age account of living with a disease, but also a journey of getting to understand cancer better. It provides insight to medical and scientific research that successfully manages to strip away the ongoing fear and misunderstanding that has commonly been associated with cancer. I will forever be indebted to the centres of medical excellence as well as my very own parents who ceaselessly continued to unearth solutions despite the path being unclear at certain points. It's important to cherish life as it is extremely fragile and tomorrow may not always be guaranteed.

Calvin dos Santos - July 2020

PART 1:

Our family's journey in search of healing for Calvin. It is a story about anguish, fear, hope, love and faith. Dedicated to the special people who supported us through this amazing journey, without them none of what is to follow would have been possible.

The Beginning

It is an unusually cool and rainy summer's day on 3rd July 2013, Charlene and I are gazing up at the chapel's ceiling that is adorned with a decorative 'swastika' pattern, both of us are in an incredibly emotional state but somehow we don't feel despaired or alone. Although we are thousands of miles away from home and in a foreign country we feel the presence of everyone's thoughts, prayers and well wishes. This space in time is the culmination of years of living in doubt, not knowing who to trust or who to believe. Now we were facing our own fears and doubts while inwardly praying for the deliverance that we had sought for such a long time. Our son Calvin was fighting for his life and we felt like ringside spectators, committed to the cause but not able to be involved at this crucial point. But to start the story here may not be enough to convey our exceptional journey; we need to start at the beginning.

But where do we begin? Ok, maybe not quite at the beginning, let's rather start from the time when Calvin began to show that there was something going wrong internally with him. It was late winter 2010, the Soccer World Cup in South Africa had just finished and we were planning a business trip to Paris so that we could attend a trade show there. As you can imagine juggling kids and work is never easy, especially when you're about to leave on a two week trip abroad. While Charlene and I poured our energy into this long overdue trip, Calvin came up with a 'mystery' pain in his stomach. The pain was such that he was unable to stand up straight and was genuinely suffering from something. Charlene being ever pro-active arranged for Calvin to see our local doctor for a medical check-up.

The check-up was there to ensure that we knew what was going on and specifically to rule out anything serious with the view that should he receive medication then Charlene's mom Ethne would be able to medicate him while we were away. The check-up produced more questions and the doctor suggested that we should go for a MRI scan at the Donald Gordon Clinic. I remember that day as clear as daylight, there I was with Calvin at the Radiology department not really knowing what to expect, but being an optimist I was not too worried, he was a 'healthy' young boy after all. After the MRI scan the doctor suggested we do an ultrasound as a precautionary scan. We then met Charlene and her mom at reception and waited for the doctor to inform us of their findings.

After a lengthy wait the doctor materialised and there at the small reception area he began with his deliberation. In his opinion Calvin was suffering from faecal impact in his stomach, in other words whatever he had eaten previously had stagnated in his stomach causing him much discomfort. There and then like any 'good' parent I thought "that is the end of his junk food binges, from now on he will only eat healthy wholesome food that is natural to human beings". I felt vindicated as I had always harboured food issues of my own, now was the time to address this issue on a family level, this was a simple solution in my 'naive' mind. The doctor went on to explain that the scan had also picked up an 'inflamed lymphatic node' in his lower abdomen, but that this was not out of place as his body was dealing with an internal crisis. In his opinion there was nothing much that we could do other than to put him on strong laxatives and change his diet so that he could pass that internal blockage naturally. We breathed a collective sigh of relief and went back home with a plan to improve Calvin's condition.

Two days later we were in a summery Paris away from our kids, somehow being on the other side of the world gave us space to think and we felt that something was amiss. However, the regular phone calls back home were enough to give us a sense that he was back on the road to recovery, at least he was starting to realise the value of eating fruit, I thought. We returned back home after our time away and were happy to see our boys as much as they were happy to see us. Our younger son Caleb latched himself onto Charlene, Calvin onto me and then vice-versa; nothing was as special as this unconditional show of love, the boys had missed us. From the corner of my eye I saw the happiness in Charlene's parents' faces, but theirs was the happiness from the relief of the burden of having to look after our beloved brats and I didn't blame them one bit. The main thing was that they were happy and Calvin had recovered fully, his recovery was credited to Ethne's untiring efforts to follow doctor's orders. We thought or at least I thought the worst was behind us, it was time to regain health at home.

It was late summer in 2010 and Calvin was finishing his soccer season at the club and preparing for final exams. He has always been a conscientious scholar and he focussed his energy into the task of passing the year. Calvin in our opinion was getting more anxious, but we thought this was natural and would pass after his exams. As his exams finished the soccer club circulated notices regarding an upcoming tour to the UK in the following year during the winter holidays. Since Calvin had followed his older cousins at the soccer club, this opportunity was not going to pass him by as his cousins had been on tour the preceding years. All that he had to do was to attend a December and January selection phase and obviously us as parents had to show our intent by putting down a deposit. He also had to promise us that schoolwork still came first and additional training would not interfere. The kids at the club were extremely talented, but this did not hold Calvin back from trying, he wanted to go on tour. In that period Calvin worked extremely hard, he respected his coaches and he juggled his schoolwork. However, he was starting to suffer from strange 'shakes and sugar-crashes', this we attributed to his physical exertions on the soccer field.

Winter 2011 came around and Calvin was selected into the 2nd touring side, they were the developmental team. We were all excited about the prospect of him touring the UK; Calvin had managed to uphold his end of the bargain and he deserved every bit of that experience. I went along as a part of a small parent contingent and was also looking forward to see my sister Suzana and her family who lived near to where we were staying. The young players were accommodated at the old Royal Holloway castle in Surrey and the parents went into more modern student accommodation. The tournament was a hive of activity with boys and girls representing different countries from around the world. The 2nd team boys faced some stiff opposition, but they were not expected to win anything, winning was for the 1st team. Over a period of a week the boys played a soccer match in the morning followed by long training sessions and then trips around London on days off. They mingled with kids from other countries; Calvin made friends with a Moroccan boy called Simon, who as fate would have it was the best player in the Moroccan side. Their first match was disastrous; they played a UK side who had won the previous year and who were intent on winning by a large margin. For my part I wasn't stressed at all as Calvin was assigned as reserve and I feared he would stay on the side line for the rest of the tour, saving me from the embarrassment of further losses. Into the second half and one of our defensive players got injured and Calvin was pushed into action. I recalled that this was an extremely muggy day, not at all great for anyone with health issues, let alone staring a bigger and better opponent. In a short break during the match Calvin was in distress, he had a very bad migraine; all I could offer was encouragement and water. Calvin pushed past his pain and did admirably, so much so that his coach took notice and from then onwards he never sat on the side-lines. They lost that first match by a huge margin, but they never despaired, from here onwards they never lost a match and in the end met their much fancied 1st team in the plate final. But before that match, in the semi-final he faced Simon his new Moroccan friend who duly scored two quick goals. Calvin's side rallied and it was not long before they equalised and in the dying minutes of some exciting play by both teams, the Moroccan goalie fumbled a tame ball that slipped between his legs and the young second string South African's were through to the finals. I could see the pain in Simon's face after they lost, but was happy to see that Calvin stuck his hand out to congratulate him on his effort. Calvin later told me that he felt sorry for him as he was such a good player. The final was an all-South African affair, the 1st team won the plate, but best of all the 2nd team had done better than expected and won runner-up medals. Calvin was all happiness and smiles. We enjoyed two more glorious days in London on our own and visited our family and did some shopping for the family back home. In retrospect we put Calvin's body through quite a lot and we were lucky that none of the more serious symptoms made an appearance during that tour. From this experience Calvin showed that for what he lacked in talent he made up in perseverance and determination, attributes that he was going to need in his not too distant future.

A Troubled Horizon

After this amazing experience we slipped back into our day-to-day existence. By the end of 2011 Calvin's soccer skills were in an upward trajectory, however on a few occasions he developed energy issues that resulted in severe shaking, vomiting and paleness. These spells happened both at club and school soccer, even prompting the school coach to lecture us as parents on what he thought adequate nutrition was all about. We weren't stupid, we knew something was not right and we started to suspect that he may have issues related to diabetes since I was one. By early 2012 when school started again Calvin was to swim at the school swimming gala. It wasn't long into that morning when Charlene got a call from the school that Calvin was very sick. I got a call at work to pick him up at the sick bay and to take him home while Charlene sorted some work issues out and booked the all-important appointment with our local doctor. As I arrived at school my thoughts wondered as to the possibilities of his affliction, I felt helpless. There he lay in sick bay, as pale as a sheet with dark rings under his eyes with a faint whiff of vomit hanging in the air, he was not well. I took him home and on the way he explained to me how after exerting himself at the swimming pool that he suddenly felt nausea, started to shake uncontrollably and eventually vomited. We went through the motions of verifying if he had eaten enough breakfast to sustain himself during the day and we joked how Charlene had made a special energising breakfast with enough carbohydrate and protein to sustain a small soccer team. Essentially it seemed to me that he had indeed consumed enough nutrition to support him on that day, something else was out-of-place. As soon as he arrived home, I had him take a shower while I made him a toasted sandwich and tea. Once he had washed up and eaten his colour returned and he looked none the worse for wear. I left soon after that to get back to work whilst Charlene took him to see the doctor. Once again the results from all the vital sign tests were normal; the doctor tried her best to explain the possibilities to Charlene. We were dumfounded, but we accepted our learned practitioner's explanations. After all who were we to doubt their expertise?

As 2012 progressed, Calvin started to lose weight at an alarming rate, but so too his height increased. It wasn't long before he had reeled in some of the taller soccer players in his team and I even had numerous parents enquire about his sudden growth spurt, especially seeing that we were a family of 'shorties'. We were not too concerned as we knew that hormonal changes were at work since he was getting into his teens, essentially his body weight was being displaced by his body height. Calvin also started to play tennis and his new love for golf started to blossom, this was to be the start of a new obsession and I was only too happy to share this with him. By the winter of 2012 Calvin's soccer season picked up pace and training sessions got tougher. During one of these sessions Calvin was in trouble, battling exhaustion during an extremely cold evening he bravely fought off waves of nausea until his body could no more. Vomiting was inevitable and he dashed away from his team and coaches in search of me. Once he saw me he burst into tears and I bundled him into my car for the long ride home. He vomited some more along the way, soiling my car door both inside and out. Once at home I tested his blood sugar with my glucose meter and was shocked to find his blood sugar hovering at 20 mmol/l (normal being anything between 4-7 mmol/l). I immediately rushed him to Sandton Clinic that night and he was admitted to the emergency ward for observation. At midnight a doctor eventually materialised with a spreadsheet and a good explanation as to what had possibly happened. My fear was that he was suffering from diabetes, but his blood sugar reading had plummeted to a very normal 5 mmol/l and all his other readings were great. The doctor's explanation was that Calvin had been exhausted by his training routine, gotten ill and his brain to counteract the low blood sugar had utilised sugar secreted from the liver as a back-up (that was when I had done the test), however after some time the insulin in the pancreas had done its work and stabilised his blood sugar. There we were driving in the early hours of a winter's morning, Calvin was fast asleep in the back of the car while I was left wondering if he was just going to suffer like this for the rest of his life. We had no answers; in fact we had no questions.

By the end of 2012 Calvin's golf took prominence in his life, he took a membership at Parkview Golf Club and did the customary club induction on his own. I was very proud that he did this all on his own as golf did teach him some valuable life lessons. Calvin's school year ended on a high note with his ongoing school achievement and to reward his hard work we promised him that he could spend a week during the December holidays with his grandparents and cousins at the family holiday house in Marloth Park which borders the famous Kruger National Park. The cherry on the top of this cake, however, was that they would attend the Alfred Dunhill European Golf Tour Championship taking place at nearby Leopard Creek. What else could a young boy with a golf obsession want from life? He was in seventh heaven and enjoyed every day of the tournament and continued to talk about his experience long after that. The only blemish to his holiday was that he got ill again while playing tennis with his cousins. Charlene's mom Ethne even spoke to me regarding this issue and the possible causes. I could not offer a proper answer as I knew very little of what was going on, but I appreciated her concern and she was right, something was wrong.

The beginning of 2013 had arrived and we celebrated by going on a golf holiday. We headed out to Prince's Grant on the KwaZulu Natal coast, the place where my own golf affliction had started, courtesy of my in-laws. This time around, however, I had a golf buddy and boy was he impressed. We crowned our holiday by playing at Port Shepstone Country Club and went back home with that internal golf monster momentarily satisfied. We went back to work, Calvin started Grade.7 and Caleb started Grade.1 at his new school. We were more worried about Caleb this time around as he had had a terrible experience at his previous school the year before. But our worries were laid to rest as Caleb took to the school and has never looked back. At least, to my mind Charlene had persevered by going against many medical professionals' best recommendations and achieved something positive and drug free for Caleb. Calvin started school with the customary swimming gala and we were going to be prepared this time around. But alas, this was not to be as we got the dreaded phone call once again. He got sick again and Charlene duly took him to the local doctor who suggested we do more blood tests and a long period glucose test. All the tests if not being inconclusive came back negative; one of the labs was even doubted if they could actually do a simple blood test, resulting in us doing secondary blood tests at another lab. By the end of March 2013 we were off to Sun City for a long weekend in the sun and a chance to play golf at the Lost City course. It was also our opportunity to catch up with our friends Tanja, Joerg and their boy Florian. After our amazing round of golf in the company of another golfer who was a regular visitor to the course we were invited for drinks with his wife. It was a kind gesture and we accepted the offer, but Calvin was struggling with a migraine and looked incredibly pale. Thankfully, when Charlene saw him she dispensed the customary pain killers with dollops of love and encouragement and in so doing he 'bounced-back' in no time. The next morning Joerg joined me for my customary early morning run around the Gary Player Golf Course. He was nursing a soccer injury on his thigh, but little did he know at the time that he was not injured but actually had a very large tumour inside his leg.

The Confirming Diagnosis
Easter 2013 came around and we were busy with our boys' birthdays as they are within days of each other. My sister Suzana and her family were also out from the UK and we were going away with my side of the family for a little time together. But this period quickly passed and my sister was back in the UK after two weeks in the African sun. As fate would have it we were invited to share a weekend away with our friends Tanja, Joerg and their son Florian at a game farm. We were told that it was going to be a fairly basic weekend in the bush, but I was secretly relishing the opportunity to roughen things up a bit. The game farm actually turned out to be fairly decent, the only inconvenience was that we had to share a large army tent as sleeping quarters. The moonlight on the first night was spectacular and there was a sense of one being so small in the scale of nature's beauty. The kids en-

joyed their night together in the bush as much as the adults enjoyed each other's company. The morning was bright and we were taken to the farm's sable antelope camp to watch the camp manager feed them. We spent quite some time in awe of these special animals, before they tired of us and their food and ambled away. We had also taken our bikes along for the dirt roads and I was keen to do some running of my own. Joerg was not coming along as his leg was still 'injured', but we soon left with the boys racing up the hill away from us. In the distance about halfway up a long winding sand road Calvin came to an abrupt stop, with Florian moving further away from him in his quest to get to the top of the hill first. I was pushing Caleb on his small bike, but kept my eye on Calvin who at this time was doubled over in the obvious vomiting position. As I got close to him I saw the all too familiar symptoms again, pale face, nausea, trembling and lack of energy. We were flummoxed, whatever he was suffering from was making life debilitating for him. Later that night we chatted with our friends as to his illness, they were shocked to hear how long this had been going on for and kindly suggested that we seek a second opinion or perhaps even see a specialist. Charlene and I decided right there and then that we needed a specialist to see Calvin; an endocrinologist was proposed as the obvious choice since his hormones seemed at odds. Charlene put pressure on the doctor to get an appointment with the specialist and a day later the doctor had forgotten to make that appointment. Charlene made the doctor make amends by getting an appointment for the end of the week. By the end of the week Charlene took Calvin to see Dr. Segal, a paediatric endocrinologist. After his first appointment Calvin had blood drawn and was given a 24 hour urine test bottle. It was also suggested we see a cardiologist and my first impression was that this was just going to be more of a time and money wasting exercise, but we complied.

Late on a May afternoon Calvin was getting an ultrasound done by the cardiologist, his concern was evident and at that point he took Charlene aside and asked that Calvin get a CT scan the next day. The next day dawned and while on the way to drop Caleb at school my phone rang and on the line was Dr. Segal, my immediate thought was that doctors never call at this time unless there is a life and death situation. "Mr. Dos Santos, we have tested your son's blood and it has come up as positive that he has an adrenal tumour, can you please complete Calvin's urine test and see me as soon as possible". I was in disbelief, I called Charlene immediately but she had also spoken to Dr. Segal and knew even more than what I knew at the time. I proceeded to work numbed in disbelief; suddenly nothing else mattered on this earth. I also had no idea where one's adrenaline glands are and the first thing I did was to 'Google' the topic and get a perspective of where the invader might be. Our next medical instruction was to take Calvin to get a MIBG (nuclear medicine) scan done; he would get an injection in his veins with radioactive imaging fluid. I recall while we were waiting for the scan we were asked to let a small boy and his granny to go in front of us. The little boy who was about four years old was in extreme abdominal pain and we were told that he was suffering from stomach cancer. I suddenly had a new perspective on what we were going through and the realisation was that there are always people in a worse-off position than ourselves, in other words accept our fate, as it could be way worse.

The following week we were in Dr. Segal's rooms once again, this time we were going to get the verdict. According to the scan Calvin had a large adrenal tumour the size of your fist known as a 'pheochromocytoma', it was situated between his kidneys and spinal column, an area with many vital organs and blood vessels. As it turns out adrenal tumours are extremely rare and even rarer in children and are genetically predisposed. The only treatment was open surgery and in South Africa there seemed to be little knowledge and expertise regarding the extraction of such a tumour. However, a 'pheo' had a 90% probability of being benign, but essentially it was an active supersized adrenal gland spewing out huge amounts of catecholamines or adrenal hormones which caused all the symptoms that he had previously suffered from.

This tumour was referred to as a 'ticking-time-bomb'. At least we had an answer and we felt somewhat empowered. Friends rallied around us and to my growing distress flowers started to arrive as fast as food hampers arrived, if I wasn't going to die from a pollen overload I stood a good chance to be buried under the load of food squashed in our swollen fridge. But we had an opportunity to see the kindness of heart displayed by so many well-wishers, everything was given unconditionally and love poured out from everywhere, it was palpable. Charlene also got a chance to repair a broken relationship with her older sister Loretta and they never looked back after that moment, love was stronger than anything else between them. We were careful in those early days to break the news to Calvin, systematically we used words such as 'growth' as opposed to tumour to explain his condition, as there was no need to get him unduly worried as he was still attending school.

More Bad News
It's amazing that in the face of disaster one can find peace and happiness. I found that I had patience beyond belief when it came to help Calvin with his homework and other tasks, but I suspected that I was trying to compensate for lost time. I wanted to spend as much time with him as possible and made sure that he did not go to bed before I had a chance to tuck him in. The doctor arranged for a more conclusive CT scan before an operation was scheduled and later the following week Charlene took him along. By this time school attendance was haphazard as he had started a drug blockade against the adrenal hormones prior to surgery and Dr. Segal suggested that Calvin would only realistically go back to school the following year. By Friday the doctor called Charlene and told her the bad news following the results of the CT scan. The tumour now was classed as a 'paraganglioma' or an extra-adrenal tumour with metastases, in other words it was cancerous. There was also a possibility that the liver was implicated, but the spleen was definitely going to be removed. This news was the

lowest point in our anguish; we spent the following nights walking around sobbing uncontrollably and even on occasion getting into bed next to Calvin who was heavily sedated just to feel him in our arms again. I found myself driving to work or even running in the morning with tears streaming down my face, Charlene was also struggling together with her family. I also knew my family was wrestling with the news and I found it extremely difficult to speak to them without being emotional.

Hell was a place that we got to know, we grew numb with our own fears. In the meanwhile we considered our options in terms of surgeons or centres of excellence in South Africa, but very little seemed on offer that could help Calvin. Eventually we narrowed the choice down to two surgeons, one an older experienced doctor and the other a young professional that oozed confidence but lacked the experience in removing this particular type of tumour. The older doctor unfortunately had some bad press in terms of medical malpractice and this was eventually confirmed many years later when he hit the headlines for all the wrong reasons – in retrospect we are thankful that we were overly-cautious. After some serious and at times exhausting 'homework' we accepted to meet the young doctor. The meeting was literally our last straw to help Calvin, but the young doctor seemed so precise and confident that we quickly accepted the plan for Calvin's surgery. In the young doctor's opinion Calvin had a large tumour that could only be removed through open surgery, however, they would only "de-bulk" the tumour as there was a real danger of severing a major blood vessel that the tumour encased. He explained that they would have to push Calvin's organs aside to enable them to get to the tumour to perform the de-bulking operation. On his team he had a liver specialist to attend to the liver and the spleen as these organs in their opinion were affected by the tumour. Also on the team were going to be two anaesthetists' and another specialist surgeon. After surgery Calvin would have to spend five days in ICU on strong sedatives and thereafter he would go into the ward to start a nuclear medicine attack on the remainder of the tumour. This would go on until the tumour had essentially shrunk and then plans to operate again to remove the shrunken tissue would be put into place. We could then appreciate why Dr. Segal had suggested that Calvin only go back to school the following year. To us this plan seemed realistic and the only real chance for Calvin to be rid of this tumour. We settled on the date for surgery, it was to be done on the 24th June.

A Small Ray Of Hope Beckons

After that appointment while driving to work my phone rang, it was our friend Tanja enquiring about our appointment. I quickly told her of our plan and I sensed that she was disappointed with our choice. She insisted that we look at the German option that she had investigated as she was not convinced that the local doctors could do this procedure as well as the Germans. I tried to allay her fears by saying that we had made up our minds and that the surgical team was excellent by South African standards. It wasn't long after her call that her husband Joerg called to say that he had forwarded us a medical paper written by a specialist doctor in Germany regarding these types of tumours and if anything else before we commit that we read this paper. To be honest nothing they said made a difference in me, I had grabbed the last remaining straw and I was unwilling to relinquish it. Going all the way to Germany was not an option for us, being so far away from home without family support and a very sick child did not seem to be an attractive option at the time. That day was one of the first days in our ordeal that I could actually focus on my work, but while doing my email responses I saw the medical paper that our friends wanted us to read. Out of respect to them I obliged and read the 150 page document which was written in English. Being an academic I had up until now read as much as I could on the topic in medical journals. The first thing that struck me was the date, this was the most recent paper I had read and it was published in 2012. Secondly it was co-authored by many medical professionals from around the world which included, German,

American and Italian doctors. Thirdly this paper was specifically aimed at patients and their families and therefore it was easy to read. All I can say is that my socks were blown off; these guys whoever they were knew their subject. I read the pertinent information first and was amazed to find that the authors spoke in terms such as "minimally invasive" surgery, "mostly benign" tumours irrespective of diagnoses especially at centres with little experience and a "full and quick" recovery after surgery. I had work to do, so I put the paper in my bag to read later at home and sent Joerg a SMS to say that the paper was the best I had read.

As soon as I arrived home that night I pulled out a highlighter to mark all the pertinent information, however I still did not fully understand what was being said. I saw images of people with huge abdominal scars who had undergone open surgery and there were images of people with tiny scars on their backs from endoscopic surgery. The authors also mentioned that open surgery was only reserved for extreme cases and that in most cases "minimally-invasive endoscopic surgery" was the only way to go. The benefits that they described included a quick recovery, 100% tumour removal and minimal scarring. Charlene then drew my attention to a letter that Joerg and Tanja had sent to us and we started to read the letter together. The letter floored us, in it our friends were pleading that we do everything possible for our son, in their eyes Calvin was part of their family and we had a responsibility to consider the best treatment that we could possibly get even if it meant travelling to another country. Well, what can one do in the face of such attractive odds but to comply wholeheartedly? Charlene and I spent the rest of the evening marvelling at the YouTube clips where the surgical team under the guidance of Prof. Walz performed endoscopic operations on patients. They looked like a jovial and relaxed bunch, even timing their procedures to perfection. We felt like we were reborn, our friends had played their part in saving our boy's life and we were indebted to them. I think we only got to bed after midnight, but sleep came easy for both of us as we knew that we were onto something good.

The following day heralded our first communication with the German doctors, Joerg had already initiated dialogue with Prof. Neumann the endocrinologist from Freiburg. Amazingly this was done whilst he was in Hungary on holiday with his family. This doctor was to become the next special person who would enter our lives with a gracious and humorous flourish. In the meantime it was the surgeon Prof. Walz from the Huyssens Stifftung in Essen who initiated the dialogue and Charlene spoke to him later that evening. It was evident from Charlene's account that Prof. Walz was extremely knowledgeable and he assured Charlene that the tumour was indeed benign and was separated from the other organs. He had the scans already on hand as our friends had ensured that he receive them for further diagnosis. In his opinion his surgical team was unique in the world because they offered the option for minimally-invasive endoscopic surgery that would remove 100% of the tumour safely. This news was a further breath of fresh air to us; we were also instructed to email all Calvin's blood pressure and heart rate results daily so that he could modulate his medication intake. Astoundingly there was no talk of charging for this service as we had been accustomed to this 'modus operandi' from our dealings with most South African doctors. As promised Prof. Walz responded every day to our emails and offered his opinion on concerns that we were experiencing.

Another friend of ours Lora in the meantime had pursued other avenues to help our cause. She had got into contact with Allen Wilson from Ireland who was part of a support group for people suffering from pheochromocytomas and paragangliomas. The support group is known as the "Pheoparatroopers" and we wasted no time in taking up the offer to make contact with Allen. We duly met Allen on Skype and chatted for over an hour. He explained his own personal journey, how as a young man he battled with depression and other more psychological issues. Doctors had no answers for him, they just provided more medication and he battled to maintain personal relationships due to the misdiagnosis. Eventually when he was diagnosed correctly he too ran into difficulties trying to find the appropriate expertise in dealing with this tumour. His own research led him to the NICHD centre in the US where he had a very large pheochromocytoma removed through open surgery and it took him roughly six months to recover, in particular detoxifying from the alpha and beta blockers seemed his biggest challenge. Allen was very aware of the German doctors, but in his opinion he thought that they would be out of our league in terms of cost as we hailed from Africa and our currency was weak. I silently thought to myself that Allen had no clue as to how much our medical aid actually cost us, South Africans fork out a lot of money to maintain basic medical services and our hospital costs are among the highest in the world. Our Skype feed was excellent that day and I could see that Allen looked particularly well, I even estimated his age to myself at around the late thirties. To our surprise he said that he was about to celebrate his fiftieth birthday and I asked how he maintained this healthful appearance. His response was simple; he abided by the principles of the Gerson and Hippocrates diets and as such had maintained his health and had no tumour recurrence since his operation. That was admirable as the Gerson diet is possibly one of the toughest diets to follow as it is meant primarily to treat 'no-hope' cancer patients. But he was living proof that there were survivors and a community existed to support each other through their own personal ordeals.

Getting The Ball Rolling
As the puzzle pieces started to fall into place we made our intention clear to the German doctors that we wanted to have the surgery done in Germany. We also needed to notify the young local surgeon and his team that we were not going forward with our intended plan. I tried to call the doctor directly but instead the receptionist acting as 'gate-keeper' fielded my call and matter-of-factly told me the doctor was very busy and that he would get back to me regarding our intention. I never received that call, but I knew that he got the message. I started to realise at

that point that some South African doctors are untouchable and one would only be able to deal with their assigned 'gate-keepers'. On the other hand the German doctors had no 'gate-keepers' and were exceptionally easy to contact regardless of the distance that separated us. The first time I called Prof. Neumann he was still on holiday but none-the-less still took my call and immediately referred to Charlene as "the lovely Mrs. Dos Santos". I immediately knew that Charlene would love this gentlemanly approach, something that is lost in our post-modern society, it was a refreshingly old fashioned approach and even I was amused by this.

At some point we needed to sort out finances and a plan in terms of our trip to Germany. It seemed like we were going to struggle to arrange the trip as we were required to visit two cities in different parts of Germany, coupled with the very busy itinerary of the two lead doctors. But we needn't of worried as Prof. Neumann had this all covered, he duly provided us with a rough itinerary that suited both the doctors and an estimate on the costs. I must say that right from the beginning since finding out what Calvin had there was no question, we would spend all we could to heal him, this I believe is every loving parent's responsibility. Thankfully, we were in a fortunate position to have an adequate medical aid cover that could be tapped for the occasion. Charlene's friend Henriette who represented our medical aid company, took over all our medical aid paperwork and on our behalf followed up every lead that eventually resulted in us being granted the go-ahead for the procedure in Germany. We would be able to at least claim back the greater proportion of the surgical bill. Henriette's assistance took much off our shoulders and allowed us to focus on other more pressing issues. Charlene was also required to apply for an emergency visa from the German consulate as she did not have an EU passport like myself and Calvin. Prof. Neumann provided the required letter and a two year visa was granted at no charge. But while sitting in the small reception area there was a poster proclaiming "Germany, land of imagination". That was as good an omen that we needed at the time and we had no doubts about this claim. Our friend Tanja took care of our flights through her travel company and got us bookings during a very busy European summer holiday season. We were ready to go.

On Wednesday the 26th June we were sadly dropping off our youngest boy Caleb (and our dogs) in Bethal, he was to spend his winter holiday with his grandparents. This included the usual family holiday at Marloth Park with his cousins and a weekend at Charlene's sister Loretta's trout farm Torbun-Le. At least we knew that he would be with family and that our time away would be more bearable for him. I admired his bravery, but he knew that his brother was not well and that we were all required to work together. Caleb had also given Calvin a card that he had made and in it was a picture of Calvin on a bed with an angel with arms outstretched above him. Caleb said that it was an angel that would protect Calvin in his "holy-bubble" and Calvin duly treasured that card. We arrived back home in time to have a shower and go over some of our trip details. While we waited for Charlene's sister Loretta to pick us up for our lift to the Gautrain station, I suddenly reflected on our situation. I looked at Charlene and said that we actually did not know what we were getting ourselves into, but that we were simply going in faith.

The flight to Zurich was uneventful; we followed Prof. Neumann's instructions for the trip. These included that Calvin be seated comfortably, no added pressure and weight on his abdomen and his last bit seemed a bit ominous but it went something like this "let's hope and pray that the tumour is silent during the trip". We were to later find out what this request actually meant. We landed on a chilly Thursday morning at around 7:00 and proceeded out of the terminal and into the train station for our trip to Freiburg in Germany. The walk for Calvin was excruciating, he was in pain and his legs were cramping badly as result of his medication. We made slow progress onto the platform and he collapsed his head on Charlene's lap and tried to regain some strength for the imminent train ride. Charlene and I looked at one another helplessly, coming so far for us to fail was not our intention, and we knew that we had to slog out the next few days prior to his surgery. Eventually the train materialised and soon we were travelling at high speeds towards Freiburg that is on the border between Switzerland and Germany. We allowed ourselves the simple pleasure of taking in the beautiful green scenery slipping past our fast-moving train.

Germany At Last
We arrived at around 10:00 in a rain soaked Freiburg and took the first taxi to the hotel that Prof. Neumann had booked for us. After dropping off our bags we decided to walk to the Freiburg University hospital and try to find the kind professor's office. We were only supposed to meet him on the following day, but at least we had some time to orientate ourselves in this beautiful university city. We also were carrying vials of Caleb's blood that were required for the family genetic testing. As it turned out the campus and hospital was enormous, and finding Prof. Neumann was going to be a challenge for freshly arrived South Africans with limited knowledge of the German language. The campus was abuzz with many students on bicycles whizzing past us and the grounds were immaculate with flowers everywhere. We eventually found the hospital reception and Prof. Neumann was summoned to meet us. It wasn't long before he materialised and it was Charlene that recognised him from his internet picture. He immediately made a bee-line towards us and said "it's a pleasure to meet the lovely Mrs. Dos Santos" whilst shaking her hand. He then turned to Calvin and said "ahh, Calvin and how are you?" Eventually he turned to me and said "it's a pleasure to meet you Mr. Dos Santos", no terms of endearment for me. We followed the professor in the rain towards his office whilst dodging bicycles (which he humorously called the "silent-death") and he said that he was happy that we had arrived earlier so that he could start some of the tests immediately.

Prof. Neumann we observed is an energetic person who never

failed to be gracious in his dealings with the people around him. It was also evident that he enjoyed the respect of his colleagues. He quickly arranged for the tests to be done earlier and from there onwards we had a good insight into the efficiency of the German medical personnel. Just about everyone spoke some English and we never waited longer than five minutes for any of the required tests. By 12:00 all the tests were done, all that remained was for Calvin to do the dreaded 24 hour urine test again, together with a 24 hour portable blood pressure monitor to measure his overall blood pressure profile. Charlene and I had our own blood drawn by Prof. Neumann for the obligatory genetic testing. After this we were ready to go back to the hotel and Prof. Neumann turned to Calvin and asked him "do you play tip-kick?" Calvin looked at me as if trying to find the answer in my face, but I was just as puzzled as he was. Prof. Neumann then explained that it was a soccer board game and that we should go with him to his house to get it for Calvin. We objected as we felt we had taken much of his valuable time but he resisted our protest. It wasn't long before we were travelling in his car heading towards his house on the outskirts of Freiburg. At his house we walked up the sloping path adorned with rosebushes leading to a pretty white Germanic-styled house and before going in his housekeeper greeted us with a friendly smile. Inside his house we waited in the dining room drinking fizzy apple juice whilst he disappeared to get the board game. While we waited there we admired his sloping back garden and noticed his twig bird feeder that reminded us of our own bird feeder at home and the ones we also love in the bush at Marloth Park. He seemed to be a man of very simple pleasures, quite similar to our own. A while later he appeared a little disappointed as he failed to find the board game. We then chatted for a while and before long the housekeeper appeared with the game which made the professor immensely happy.

After the professor dropped us off at our hotel we had a chance to unpack and shower in our room. The room was comfortable and in an alcove in the wall was a small statue of Buddha. Our hotel was not a typical German establishment, it had more of an Eastern feel, but what the restaurant served was really impressive. It catered for mainly a younger clientele and mostly people who were there to deal with the university. They had an extensive vegetarian menu which was unlike the meat, potatoes and bread meals that I had expected. Our first meal funnily enough consisted of falafel balls in a bed of couscous with a fresh salad which Calvin really enjoyed. As it was summer the daytime light extended deep into the night and we found ourselves exploring the centre of Freiburg to sort out our communication devices. We enjoyed walking around the neat city that is surrounded by the fringes of the Black Forest and when we looked a little lost a couple immediately approached us to help us find our bearings. We had also noticed that the regular bell that tolled in the city came from the impressive Freiburg cathedral that we wanted to visit when we had some more time on hand. The evening eventually came and we had our meal in the restaurant before collapsing in bed from exhaustion. The only issue that Calvin had to contend with was his blood pressure monitor that kept constricting his arm every half an hour to monitor his overall blood pressure.

The next morning we had arranged to meet the professor at 9:00 to carry on with the remainder of the tests for Calvin. It wasn't long before we had finished and the professor announced that we were to meet his wife for lunch in the countryside. He also told us since he did not require us to be in Freiburg on Saturday and Sunday he had taken the liberty to book us into a "gasthaus" owned by a dear friend of his in the Black Forest and that was where lunch was going to be. We were once again travelling towards the professor's house on a very sunny late Friday morning and once there we met his serene wife Hetty. She welcomed us as if we were long lost friends and seemed to know every detail about our story. The trip to Glottertal in the Black Forest was smooth with us taking in the wonderful scenery of the German countryside in its 'summer-dress'. The professor's friend and owner of the Gasthaus Adler welcomed us warmly. This establishment was exactly what I was expecting to see in Germany, but it was even better than my expectations. It was a very traditional Germanic-styled building very similar to the English Tudor-styled buildings. The inside was decorated in everything traditional which included a lot of stuffed animals and mounted deer antlers on the walls and the furniture was made from dark stained oak. The owner and her staff were all dressed in traditional German outfits typical of that area. Our lunch consisted of baked trout encrusted with slivered almonds taken from the stream that flowed past the gasthaus and the most amazing salad made from the fresh produce in their vegetable garden. During our lunch the professor asked if we would like to attend a string quartet recital at the hospital which was for his good friend that was on dialysis and who had worked for many years for the Berlin Philharmonic Orchestra. We accepted the offer and made our way back to Freiburg while the professor spoke of his retirement public lecture (on genetics) and his farewell party. He also wished for us to be part of this occasion but was well aware of our commitment to Calvin. Charlene and I were taken aback by the gesture, especially for the fact that we already felt so at home with him and his wife even though we had just met. After a well-deserved afternoon nap we ambled towards the small hospital reception area where we met the professor, his wife, his sick friend and the other members of the quartet all of whom were young musical students. A small audience consisting mostly of friends, hospital staff and patients enjoyed the recital. We were very impressed by the professor's talent and love of classical music. We noted that his sick friend was very appreciative of the professor's simple but meaningful gift to him.

A Weekend In The Black Forest
The following morning was a rainy Saturday and we planned to visit the Freiburg Cathedral before heading out to Glottertal. The cathedral was very impressive and Charlene managed to light a few prayer candles for Calvin and his brother who was far from us. Outside in the on-off drizzle was a local produce market and soup

kitchen for the poor. We purchased some fresh assorted berries and enjoyed these while looking at the other produce. Charlene even managed to do a little clothes shopping in the city centre while I got the much needed anti-cramping salts for Calvin. Thereafter, we took a taxi to Glottertal and it wasn't long before we were lying on our beds having the much fancied afternoon nap. After our nap we took a walk around the village admiring the forest, vineyards, orchards, vegetable gardens, wheat fields and wood stacks. Everywhere we looked was picture perfect, but most notably on every building, yard or field was the symbol of the cross. We visited the Glottertal cathedral whose bells rang out hourly; this seemed to be a key feature of all German towns. By then Calvin's legs started to cramp and we started our walk back to the hotel. As we neared the hotel one of the hotel's employees came rushing up to us and said "herr dos Santos, the professor is waiting for you!" We looked at one another slightly perplexed as we couldn't recall making any arrangements with the professor. There in the restaurant was the professor looking very relaxed and smiling. He was there to take us up to the St. Peter's in the Black Forest cathedral which was about 30 km away. We were blown over by another gesture of kindness; this man seemed to have no end to his thoughtfulness. We enjoyed the rest of the afternoon in his company while visiting the cathedral which was truly exquisite. While there we got to witness the choir in practice for their Sunday mass and the professor lit a personal prayer candle for Calvin. We then went to feed the professor's horse at the stables back in Glottertal, where he kindly insisted that Calvin do him the honour of feeding his horse. On the way back to the hotel the professor said that he and his wife would like us over for Sunday lunch and the opportunity to meet the rest of his family. We accepted the invite and looked forward to the occasion. That evening we spoke on Skype with the family back home and got a chance to speak to Caleb who was clearly missing mom and later we sat down to a silver-service dinner in the German tradition.

The following morning as Charlene and Calvin lay asleep I headed out on my usual morning run, except that this time there was nothing usual about this particular run. As I absorbed the scenery my thoughts raced back to my early, dark, cold-winter emotional runs, but now here I was running in a bright morning full of hope for Calvin's future, nothing could be better for me. The professor duly arrived to collect us after a late breakfast and soon we were heading back into Freiburg. Before going to his house he was required to collect his youngest daughter Luise that stayed during the week in a special home for the mentally handicapped. The professor had already spoken about Luise to us and whenever he spoke of her we could feel the pain that he had gone through. It made us realise that this may have attributed to the way in which he related to people, it was pure selfless love and we watched and learned from him. After collecting Luise we made our way to the professor's house where we met his other daughter Fanny and her fiancé Holger. Lunch was very relaxed and afterwards Fanny and Holger drove us back to our gasthaus in Glottertal.

On Monday morning we woke up and visited the little stores in Glottertal to buy some last minute presents. We took the taxi back to Freiburg for Calvin's last test with Prof. Neumann. This day would mark the start to the final leg of our journey as we would travel to Essen. The professor looked preoccupied when we arrived and told us that Calvin's thyroid function test results were not good but that we should not worry until after his surgery had been done. He also sensed that Calvin was apprehensive and we said that he was very scared of the surgery. He turned to Calvin and said "Calvin I will not send you to any surgeon, Prof. Walz is my friend for many years and I trust him with all my patients". Calvin accepted his point of view and seemed content for the time being. Soon after Calvin's last test we prepared ourselves to say good bye to the professor, but he would have none of it. He had the train schedules in hand and he knew exactly which train we should catch, but he also insisted on personally dropping us off at the train station. Again we protested in vain as we felt we were taking him away from his work, but he insisted. At the train station he got hold of a train official that spoke English and he arranged our travel tickets quickly and hassle free. In the meantime the professor disappeared only to reappear with four packets full of German pastries for our trip. We just couldn't believe his generosity and then it was the sad farewell. Charlene had already offered that he visit us in South Africa and he seemed very interested in the idea. He bid us farewell and promised that he would keep in contact, but most of all he wished Calvin a healthy recovery.

Our Appointment With Destiny

The Inter City Express train moves at very high speeds and makes travel a real pleasure. Five hours later we were in Essen which was definitely nothing like Freiburg. It was a flat, featureless city, but a city that held much promise for us. After finding our hotel we walked the 1.5km to the clinic. Calvin was not feeling well at all and I was secretly happy that we were walking towards our final destination. The hospital was built in the Bauhaus tradition and was opened by Hermann Goering in 1935, with three brand new wings having been opened earlier in 2013. It was also a government hospital, but nothing about it suggested that it was. We were soon pointed to one of the new wings where we were to meet Prof. Walz. It wasn't long before he appeared covered from head to toe in a turquoise surgeons outfit and vivid green rubber clogs. He introduced himself and asked that we be shown to our room so that he could have further discussions with us. We complied and walked into room no.0317, the room was tastefully decorated with state of the art equipment. Inside on the table was a tray with an assortment of cold meats, cheese and bread. Prof. Walz then entered the room and sat in a chair near to us. He directed his questions to Calvin while Charlene fired back answers. On three occasions he asked that Charlene not answer on behalf of Calvin and so Charlene got his message and remained quiet for the rest of the session. He then turned to us and said that we were welcome to stay at the hospital for the night, but that he only required for us to be there the next day at 9:00. We agreed and left to stay the night at our hotel. On the way back we spoke about our first meeting with the professor and realised that this was going to be a very different interaction.

The next morning we were waiting in the room at the hospital for the first medical professional to arrive and start Calvin's preparation for surgery. The first doctor was Prof. Groeben the anaesthetist; we dubbed him 'the saint' for his gentle demeanour. He methodically went about asking all the pertinent questions and Charlene asked about Calvin's asthma. It turned out that Prof. Groeben was an asthma specialist as well, for us getting this combination was a real miracle. Thereafter, Calvin had a battery of procedures done including, blood pressure tests, swabs, the drawing blood samples, etc. We met the assistant surgeon Dr. Judith Daimer, who also asked a number of questions. We also started to orientate ourselves in relation to what was on offer at the hospital. Calvin had worked out where to get free drinks and we were worried that he had just taken one without paying. We duly asked the nurse at reception and were told that this was part of the 'package' that we had paid for; we could help ourselves in the cafeteria whenever we wanted. Later that afternoon Prof. Walz made his next appearance and again sat down in the chair near to us. This time he was speaking directly to us as parents and I sensed that he was about to rock our 'little happy boat'. He said that Calvin had a particularly large tumour and that his colleagues were of the opinion that open surgery was the only option. But, he then said that he was against this as endoscopic surgery provided many benefits. He also mentioned that he had conceptualised how he was going to do this procedure, he would have to enter the body cavity via the two sides of his back and remove the tumour piece by piece through a vacuum bag process they referred to as "morcelisation". I appreciated his candidness but also his imagination, Germany after all was living up to being a "land of imagination".

D-Day For Calvin

'D-day' had arrived for us. It was early morning on the 3rd July when I made my way from the hotel to be on time before Calvin was moved to the surgery prep area. I had also missed breakfast as Charlene and I had decided to fast for the day. The walk in the drizzle was brisk and my thoughts went out to Calvin, today was the day after many years that he would eventually get rid of a tumour that Allen Wilson referred to as "the beast". As I walked into the room I noticed that there was a hive of activity around Calvin, he had to get dressed in the usual open backed surgery gown, a surgical nappy and had to wear ridiculously long compression stockings that had us giggle while trying to slip them on. The smiling attendant then pushed him on his bed to the surgery area, where we said our good-byes to one another. This was probably the hardest part for me and Charlene, as we had to be strong for him without breaking down in tears. We soon headed out the doors and made our way to the hospital chapel. In fact Prof. Walz suggested in jest that we go sightseeing or shopping during the surgery, but eventually he said the chapel was a good place. He also mentioned to us that on the ceiling was a remnant of Germany's history and that we should only see it as that. This hint made me slightly curious and at that moment I had a little task to complete in the sombreness of that day. We sat inside the chapel gazing up at the ceiling for our clue but we struggled to find anything remotely familiar. The era in which the hospital was constructed was at the rise of the Nazi empire and therefore a Nazi symbol was the obvious clue. Then like an optical illusion amongst the religious symbols inlaid in the chain-link pattern was the inglorious 'swastika', a cold shiver ran down my spine just observing this. But, I realised that this was just another of man's many meaningless symbols of power. The other historical fact was that Essen was heavily bombed during WW2 and very little remained of the old city, but amazingly this building was never destroyed. We spent about two hours in the chapel with Charlene being the strong one, supporting me through my periodic emotional weakness. Charlene lit some prayer candles for Calvin and eventually we walked hand-in-hand back to the room.

That day was not only important to us, but we realised that countless people back home and around the world were praying for us. People I have never met in my life carried our hopes alive on the wings of prayer. Chrissie Bell, Henriette's mom who resides in the UK and her prayer group never left our side during our ordeal. I think we may have got at least one phone call and an email each day from Chrissie to keep our focus in faith. In Johannesburg Calvin's school De La Salle Holy Cross held a special mass for healing. The amount of people besides friends and family praying for Calvin was beyond belief. In this action alone it was evident that love, faith and prayer surpassed our wildest imaginations. Just being part of this outpouring humbled us as parents. It was a simple 'formula' but I quickly realised that as humans we tend to complicate things and yet having faith at that moment was a truly uplifting experience for all involved.

That afternoon we were desperate for some news and we tried not to dwell on the possibilities. I can honestly say that open surgery started to loom large the longer the surgery took without any news being relayed back to us. Chrissie called us and said "your son is healed in Jesus name, the tumour is no more". By 13:00 the assistant surgeon Dr. Daimer popped her head into our room and announced that everything was going according to plan, Prof. Walz was still operating endoscopically. One part of the tumour had already been removed and now they were going to concentrate on the other side. Charlene and I breathed a collective sigh of relief; it was all that we needed to know at that stage. We spent the rest of the afternoon fielding emails from friends and family, and also did another trip to the chapel and the hospital's garden. We felt content by the news that everything was going as the professor had planned and that we could do no more than be there for each other. By 19:00 Dr. Daimer made her last appearance and announced that the tumour had been completely removed and that the surgeons were doing their final procedures prior to Calvin being prepared for his stay in ICU. The professor eventually made his appearance a little after that news and looked visibly drained. He looked straight at us and said "never bring your child with a tumour that size again". As Prof. Walz explained the procedure to us, Charlene out of concern offered the tired surgeon one of her sweets. It turned out to be a chocolate coated toffee which resulted in the professor almost choking on the offending gift. After the humorous moment the professor explained that after removing the main tumour the surgical team did a visual scan with their endoscopic camera to make certain that they had removed everything. In his words he said "as we did our visual scan a very small growth was highlighted and we removed it". We were in disbelief, how could 'highlights' occur inside a small body?

Living Through Intensive Care
After that discussion I left to go back to my hotel and Charlene waited to be called to ICU to see Calvin. She only got to see him at 2:00 the next morning when he started to call for her. She was a little shocked to see his state as he appeared as if he had been in a car accident. His eyes were swollen shut and the swelling over the rest of his body was extensive as a result of the very long operation. By 6:00 that morning I was back in the hospital and found Charlene on her way to the ICU and joined her. It was hard to see Calvin in that state, but he immediately recognised me and said "dad where have you been? I missed you". My knees almost buckled and I had to hold back my tears. I also felt for Charlene as she had soldiered the night on her own and here I walk into the limelight after a good night's rest. But, I guess that happens to many parents. He was extremely thirsty and wanted the yoghurt on offer as it soothed his sore throat after being intubated for so long. We fed him in bed as if he was a baby again, but we did not mind. He was also in a bit of discomfort from the surgery and complained bitterly about the urine catheter and other bits and pieces plugged into him. But these were small discomforts in

the face of what he had endured for so long. His sense of humour came to the fore when he described the first time that he was able to partly see the nurse as, "arrghh,...a pixelated lady". We all had a good laugh, not because of the joke but the fact that his sense of humour was intact. The rest of the day was spent pretty much between his bouts of sleep, our visits to the chapel and connecting with friends and family. He remained in ICU until the next day and Charlene soldiered on for another night.

The following morning as I was walking back to the hospital my cell phone rang, it was a lady with a thick English accent, I didn't get her name but she was part of Chrissie's prayer group. She said "in Jesus name your son will end his stay in ICU today, he is healed". In my disbelief I thanked her for her kindness and thought about this for the rest of the way. People were still concerned for Calvin's healing and more amazingly these were people we did not even know. It was hard to discount the power of faith in the face of what we had experienced, but again it was an extremely humbling moment. I found Charlene in ICU again, but this time Calvin had a 'problem', his stomach wanted to work. He had tried to hold back as much as he could as he was in a very compromising position and he could not work out what the process was if he needed the dreaded 'no.2'. A little unknowingly we asked the male nurse in attendance and offered to help, but he immediately said it was his job and he would come back with the "toiletten-wagen". As such a toilet on wheels appeared with the smiling nurse and he politely asked us to leave while he assisted Calvin in his need. We were blown away by the dignity shown and soon afterwards he called us back in. Calvin had been cleaned up and was now in a wheelchair as opposed to the bed so as to change his position to relieve the pressure on his back. By midday Calvin was given the 'green-light' to go back to his ward room, his stay in ICU was over.

Although Calvin had made the transition from ICU to general ward he was still in much pain and attached to a few lines, most irritatingly the urine catheter. Calvin was struggling with his breathing as he had fluid on his lungs. Apart from the retained fluid much swelling was still evident all over his body. Our mission as parents was to assist him wherever possible and to mobilise his body as instructed to reduce his swelling. This was easier said than done, it took a fair amount of massaging and limb manipulation to kick-start his mobilisation phase. We also had the weekend ahead of us to help Calvin recover to a point that we could prepare for our journey back home. Prof. Walz was off for the weekend, but ensured that members of his team were available at all times. We also got to watch how the nurses operated in this environment and were taken aback by their patience, thoughtfulness and knowledge. In one instance Calvin's pain medication made him hallucinate and we summoned the doctor on duty. After a few discussions with us and the nurse on duty, some of which was in German, Dr. Bolli turned to us and said that the nurse had a good idea. Her suggestion was that Calvin try a homeopathic pain killer that had no side effects, the young doctor had no qualms with that suggestion. We were again speechless, here we were witnessing a doctor openly accepting a nurse's suggestion regarding medication and to crown all this was that it was homeopathic. In the second instance a young nurse by the name of Sarah made her first appearance on Saturday, by that time Calvin was starting to get around a bit, but mostly in a wheelchair. She knew that he would improve quickly and that he would soon be bored with what little entertainment the hospital offered. She asked Calvin if he liked 'Playstation' to which a big encouraging smile appeared on his face. She duly brought the gaming console and arranged for it to be installed by the maintenance crew the next day. Hesitatingly Charlene thanked her and asked if the gaming console belonged to the hospital, to which she replied that it was her own and that in any case her boyfriend wasn't going to miss it. Again we were struck by simple gestures like these, we were truly being blessed.

The Disbelief Of Total Healing

As the weekend progressed Calvin made some remarkable improvements of his own. By Sunday he was walking unassisted as he had eventually rid himself of the pesky catheter and made regular trips to the chapel and garden. The weather also got into the thirties and it felt odd to be enjoying an out of season summer away from home. In all our nebulous excitement we still missed everyone back home, especially Caleb. Thankfully we connected regularly with friends and family, and it was as if they all visited us there in that room in Essen. Those 'visits' were special to us and a constant reminder of the people that supported our daily progress. Prof. Neumann had also kept contact with us to find out Calvin's progress and to relay to us any developments after the surgery. During those frequent calls he shared with us an insight about Calvin's precarious condition. In his words the danger was never going to be "organ damage", but rather "if he played a game of soccer he could die from a massive cardiac arrest" precipitated by a flood of adrenal hormones. This was a sobering thought and now I could understand his concerns over the 'behaviour' of the tumour during our flight to Germany.

Monday heralded the start of the week and one could sense that the hospital was a hive of activity once more. I was particularly interested in seeing Prof. Walz after the weekend as we needed to confirm our flight back home and only he could give us the go-ahead. At around 7:30 the professor, his colleagues and nurses came into our room. With all those people the room seemed particularly small. But I could see that the professor was in a very relaxed mood, as the jokes rolled one after each other. Our amazement at Calvin's incredible recovery was received as a very normal course of events; his quick recovery was expected by the professor. At that stage Calvin still had fairly large plasters covering his surgical wounds and so the professor proceeded to remove these in front of us. To our absolute amazement the scars were miniscule. The professor also had no qualms regarding our proposed departure date and even went as far as suggesting that Calvin go back to school as soon as possible. Jokingly he turned to

Calvin and said "I don't do this special operation for you to miss school". Later that day Prof. Neumann called us again with really good news, he had received the histology report and the tumour was confirmed as benign. After weeks of rolling bad news, we were now moving in the opposite direction and enjoying every ounce of good news.

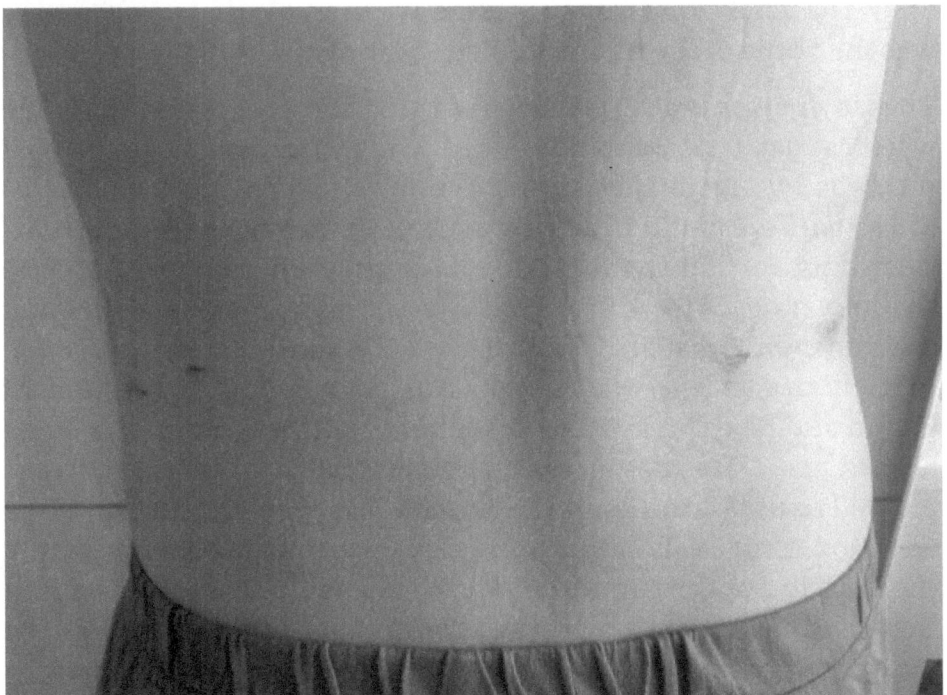

Calvin's surgery scars revealed

But Prof. Neumann was not happy with the news that we were leaving so soon. He insisted that we spend another week in Germany so that Calvin could fully recuperate. In his unique manner of speech he said to Charlene that she needed to "relax for the soul". He even went as far as to arrange a stay in a castle hotel known as "Hugenputts" that was managed by a South African lady. I must say we were very tempted by the idea, but trying to get flights in a busy holiday period proved to be very difficult. When Prof. Walz heard about this idea he again joked with us and suggested that we go home as planned and phone Prof. Neumann after we had arrived. But Charlene was having none of that idea as Prof. Neumann held a special place in her heart and she did not want to disappoint him after all he had done for us. As such Charlene called Prof. Neumann and explained our predicament with our flight and he understood our dilemma. Being always interested that we enjoyed the marvellous sights that Germany had to offer, the kind professor suggested we visit "Villa Hugel" which was the home of the infamous Krupp family.

Tuesday began as a very warm morning and progressed to be the warmest day that we experienced while in Germany. At the hospital Prof. Walz notified us that we were to do a MRI scan on Calvin so that we could provide concrete evidence to the South African doctors that the tumour was completely removed. At 9:00 that morning we were in the radiology section of the hospital and met the radiologist Prof. Koch. He was very interested in our case, particularly because the tumour was evident in the prior scan of Calvin and he expressed his disbelief that the tumour was overlooked and classed as an inflamed lymphatic node. He then explained to us how difficult the surgery had been and that on three occasions Prof. Walz called him for precise information regarding the location of the tumour from the available scans. We realised there and then that this operation was a team effort and required pin-point accuracy. After Calvin finished his scan we went back to our room just in time for lunch and started to plan our outing to Villa Hugel. It wasn't long and we were heading out of the hospital in a taxi and taking in the sights of Essen. We arrived at the gates of a large wooded estate and walked the long road towards the sumptuous palace. We enjoyed our outing immensely and it provided us with an opportunity to see if Calvin would cope with the next day's long haul back home. He seemed ready.

Homeward Bound

As I walked towards the hospital once more my suitcase wheels 'clippety-clopped' along the cobbled path I knew so well by now.

This was Wednesday 10th July and we were eventually going

home with Calvin, our mission in Germany was complete. At the hospital the staff seemed to be smiling more at us, maybe they were glad to see the back of us or they were truly happy for us. Either way we were all a happy group of people. Charlene had asked Prof. Walz that before we leave that we would like some group photographs and he obliged, even if he was a very busy surgeon. There we were all smiling at each other, making jokes and taking photographs. Our usually austere room cleaner asked in broken English if Calvin was well, to which I nodded and her face broke into a surprising smile. After that Prof. Walz took some photographs of his own of Calvin's back, we could see the pride he showed for his handiwork. In his goodbye to us he handed us the copies of the scan and confirmed that all was clear, the tumour was removed completely. He then turned to Calvin and asked him how he felt and wished him all the best in getting back to school. We were overjoyed as the knowing that Calvin was completely healed meant more to us than anything else at that moment.

We caught the ICE train for a last time and whizzed towards Frankfurt Airport while taking in the pastoral sights of the German countryside for one more time. We also ensured that we found as many pretzel stands along the way so as to satisfy our taste buds of these delectable warm and chewy snacks. I particularly enjoyed the ones encrusted with pumpkin seeds, Calvin liked the plain salted ones and I think Charlene had eyes for the sweet pastries. Anyway we were making a holiday out of our trip back home, we were still in Germany after all. Once at the airport we went about the serious business of trying to buy as many chocolates for the people back home. I'm still astounded at how many slabs of Milka-Oreo we managed to smuggle home in our bags. After the arduous task of buying armfuls of chocolates we had our last meal at the airport. This consisted of sauerkraut, sausages and pretzels washed down with ice cold beer. Calvin had a soft drink, too young to enjoy the pleasures of ice-cold beer. We were soon making our way to the designated departure gate and it wasn't long before we felt like we had arrived back home even if we were still in the airport. We heard the familiar sounds of Afrikaans, Zulu and Xhosa; we saw the sight of springbok rugby jerseys stretched over ample beer bellies and the colours of the flag on the flight attendants uniform. We were almost home.

Calvin managed remarkably well on this trip. I cannot remember him complaining about anything and he even carried his own backpack over his wounds. The flight back was uneventful and we all rested as best we could. On a chilly Thursday morning in July we touched down softly in a mist shrouded Johannesburg, we were home. After taking the Gautrain back to Sandton, Loretta collected us at the very same spot we were dropped off two weeks before and thereby completed the perfect circle of our most amazing journey. As soon as we got home we called Caleb who was still in Bethal and started to unpack. Loretta kindly did some much needed shopping for us and returned to pack our fridge. It wasn't long after Loretta eventually left when the doorbell rang for the first time, there at our door stood some of Charlene's friends who had supported us all along the way and who were extremely keen to see Calvin. They also came overloaded with food and I was once again playing 'Tetris' with food in my fridge, but it was all much appreciated. Liezl, Henriette, Celeste and Liezl's daughter Tayla made up this overjoyed welcoming party and we gladly recounted our amazing experiences to them. Out of the corner of my eye I saw Calvin standing in the garden in a hunched position and then he deftly flicked his sand-wedge towards the ball at his feet and watched as the ball eventually settled a foot away from the hole on the practice green. I knew there and then that Calvin was home and that he was going to be ok.

The Discomfort Of Being Normal

After our initial harrowing experience, both Charlene and I had learned much about this unusual disease; and to some extent so had Calvin. From being completely ignorant about this disease, we were in a position of understanding a lot more about the symptoms, the consequences and the best treatments. This we were able to do because everyone we came across contributed something towards our cause. Our knowledge was their knowledge and our experience became their experience. We could not have managed this process any other way.

The means of managing this disease are relatively simple. Firstly we understood the symptoms very well from our first-hand experience, should they ever arise. Secondly doing simple urine tests every 6 months to measure hormone levels apply preventative screening. As this disease tends to have genetic predispositions we were able to monitor Caleb as well, thankfully his test showed that he did not share the same genetic mutation. Thirdly as a family we have vowed to do the best we can to live a healthy lifestyle and that meant revisiting our diet in a responsible and sustainable manner. Happily Calvin had a urine screening test done two weeks after returning home and the results were better than what was expected as all the hormone values were well within the normal range. We also worked hard to strengthen his body for sport through biokinetics. The result was lots of power off the golf tee, even outdriving me regularly. Calvin also worked his way back into the school tennis A-team which was a real surprise for us. Since that surgery Calvin ceased to take any medication which was good for him, however the effects of the catecholamines (or adrenal hormones) still persisted for some time and it was a while before his body detoxed. The strange thing about this miraculous operation was that Calvin experienced post-trauma stress, which to some degree impaired his concentration, time and patience provided healing. Despite this issue Calvin got into the swing of school and started to engage with his work in a positive manner. More than this we could not expect, we were only too happy to see a 'normal' child again.

At that time we thought that should Calvin ever show signs of a tumour re-growth we were in a better position to do something about it, fast. We just did not know when that possibility may arise. We were also fortunate to have two world-leading professors in their fields on our side. We remained in continuous contact with each other and they remained open to supporting us here at the bottom end of Africa. So together with Dr. Segal our local endocrinologist we felt that we had the best preventative team on hand that we could trust implicitly. From a medical point of view we were always learning and we encourage that everyone who reads this story does the same. Knowledge and understanding is empowering, and having a supportive medical team on hand is comforting. And, never, ever settle for second best, even if it means going to another part of the world.

We Are Not Alone

You may ask yourself if this is a common disease and the educated answer is no. However, we have cause to believe that as the disease is so hard to detect there may be many more unaware sufferers and this is a very dangerous notion. In the month after returning from Germany we heard of three other adolescents who had the same disease. Through our local doctor we were able to forward the details of our German saviours. Sadly, another boy did not survive the ravages of this tumour and passed away on a school camp in the Drakensburg on the 16th August 2013. In his case help was too far away and our understanding of this tumour leads us to believe even if a proper rescue team arrived on time there was very little that they could do for him. According to his mother he had showed all the classic symptoms, but once again it seems that inexperienced doctors 'dropped the ball' with catastrophic results. His story is now part of our story and a constant reminder how fortunate we really are. In the darkest hour of Calvin's suffering he asked the question "why did I get this?" For any parent this is a very difficult question to answer. Now, however, he understands that he is not alone; he knows that we are all with him.

Our friend Joerg who together with his wife Tanja led us to Germany, also found themselves in a real predicament at around the same time as us. In return we were able to share the news of our experience and suggested to Joerg that South Africa may not be the best place to remove his tumour. As Joerg was already in contact with Prof. Walz, arranging his operation in Germany took a couple of emails and phone calls. Unfortunately Prof. Walz is a visceral surgeon and Joerg's tumour was not his speciality. However, he got Joerg into contact with another surgeon in Bochum who specialised in these types of tumours and the tumour was successfully removed. His recovery was swift, far shorter than suggested by his local doctor.

It was a strange coincidence that Calvin and Joerg were diagnosed with a tumour literally days from each other. They share something in common; they are fighters and survivors. Joerg shared a humorous and yet sobering take on our story. He said that "help came from above". What he was talking about was an incident earlier in the year when a helicopter was forced to land on their estate during a bad storm. On seeing the helicopter land Joerg and Florian got into their car and went to find out why it had landed and to offer some help. It turned out that the two occupants were en route to Pretoria from their game farm and were just going to sit the storm out before proceeding. Joerg invited them to his house for some drinks while the storm dissipated and they readily accepted the kind offer. Once the storm cleared they were off again and Jan extended an offer in return for Joerg's kindness that was going to be pivotal to us all. Jan who was the pilot owned a game farm in the Swartruggens area; he said to Joerg that he could visit any weekend and to bring friends with him as well. The rest as you know is history; that weekend was life changing and thus, help truly came from above.

PART 2:

After the ordeal we faced as a family in 2013, little did we know that it was just the beginning. We were about to simultaneously face our worst fears and best outcomes. Through our personal journey we once again came across incredible people that we consider to be true 'angels'. Our story of hope continues.

The Problem Is In Your Genes

It's December 2016 and I'm sitting next to Calvin on an Air France flight bound for Paris. It's just the two of us, Charlene has bravely stayed home for Caleb and entrusted Calvin's wellbeing to me. My mind is preoccupied with everything that is going to happen ahead of us, but it also drifts back to the past to find the intersection points that connect the past with the present. After Calvin's miraculous recovery due to the lifesaving operation to remove his primary tumour in Germany our family life more or less got back to normal. Calvin proceeded to finish his primary school in late 2013 with some effort on his part to catch up the schooling that he had lost in preparation for his operation in Germany. We swiftly then moved into 2014 and Calvin went into high school where he really started to find his feet. He immediately took to the different format of the school and enjoyed every part of being considered a young adult.

However, we were quickly reminded of his condition when Prof. Neumann eventually started to give feedback on some of the genetic tests that were done in Germany. His first email confirmed that Calvin had the SDHB mutation and the second email confirmed that I carried the gene and mercifully Caleb and Charlene were clear. This started the next stage on my part of trying to find out all about this gene, but more importantly I had to let my family know that they could have it too. This was easier said than done. My parents thought that the suggestion that they could have this mutation was preposterous. I could see that it hurt them, particularly my father and I certainly did not want to accuse anyone as I had my own guilt to deal with. I also informed my sisters but was acutely aware that my sister Suzana had children of her own and how this news might have impacted her world. After hearing the news Suzana called me and explained that she had discussed the issue with her husband Andrew and had decided that because no one in their family had symptoms they would choose not to do the test unless it was absolutely necessary. So we parked this matter and got on with our lives.

Not long after that episode and in consultation with my endocrinologist it was decided that I do an investigative MRI scan so as to rule out any possible connection to the gene I was carrying and my late adult onset type 1 diabetes. The scan only gave me proof that I had a brain, thankfully! However I got a taste of what Calvin gets on a routine basis and I admire his patience in these times. By August 2014 Calvin was back doing the first comprehensive scans after his surgery in Germany. At this stage Calvin had been handed over to the paediatric oncology unit at the Donald Gordon Clinic under the care of a very 'prickly' oncologist with a wide ranging reputation. In consultation with Prof. Neumann, Charlene requested that Calvin do a full body MRI scan. When the oncologist heard of this request it became apparent that our relationship was definitely planted on shaky ground. However, Charlene resisted and instructed our medical aid to approve the procedure. The scans were dutifully done and later that same day Charlene called to ask me to go past the clinic to pick up the scan report. It was a late winter afternoon but warm nonetheless when I drove up to the clinic. After collecting the scans and report I decided because the traffic was a little on the heavy side that I would wait it out in my car while I read the report. I sat riveted in my car as my eyes quickly scanned the contents of the report, my heart was literally in my mouth as I tried to make sense of what I was reading. In the report the area where the primary tumour had resided remained clear, however, two tumours were located in the vertebral column, one on the T12 and the other in the sacrum. There and then my happy world crashed around me. I drove home in quiet contemplation, wondering how I was to break the news to Charlene.

Our home in the late afternoon like other homes is a hive of activity. It's usually homework time, supper preparation and a quick catch up on each other's day. I noted that Charlene was in a relaxed mood, obviously confident that all was well, yet I struggled to break the news to her. Eventually after summoning enough courage I blurted out, "Calvin has two tumours". I watched her face slowly react and could see the disbelief in her eyes. We stood there both transfixed in the kitchen and immediately started to discuss our options. It was decided that we would be rational and the best option was to discuss the issue with our German doctors. I was actually convinced since they performed the miracle on Calvin that they would have an answer for us once again. It also dawned on us that Charlene's insistence for a full body scan actually paid off, contrary to the oncologist's recommendation. We also quickly understood why these tumours were initially undetected, firstly Calvin's primary tumour was of such a size that it demanded all the attention, but it also occluded the much smaller tumour on the T12 vertebra. Secondly, all the scans had only focused on the abdominal cavity and thus completely omitting the sacral area where the second tumour was. These were metastatic tumours that were a result of Calvin's primary tumour being undetected for so long and essentially they were pheochromocytomas located in the spine. But this knowledge we did not yet quite comprehend.

The Much Needed Doctor's Visit
Our German doctors eventually gave us news that was difficult

to accept. The issue of surgery was out of the question as these tumours resided in bone, an area of much complexity. However, the suggestion was that Calvin undergo MIBG therapy or nuclear medicine therapy. We duly started to read up on the treatment and met the nuclear medicine specialist in Johannesburg. We found out that the treatment is done through a radioactive transfusion and that the side effects are usually minimal. MIBG reportedly works well for pheochromocytomas and as such we accepted the treatment. As fate would have it earlier in the year Professor Walz, Calvin's surgeon in Germany had confirmed that he would be visiting us in Johannesburg on his way to his safari holiday. This visit was exceptionally well timed since it would be in September just before Calvin's treatment in October, encouragement was on its way.

On the 18 September 2014 Charlene and I waited in anticipation at the airport for the imminent arrival of Professor Walz and his wife Doris. We stood there jostling up between distraught family members that were waiting for survivors of the deadly church building collapse in Lagos, Nigeria. Television camera crews went about interviewing those that had made it back, while family members stood by in silence. It suddenly dawned on me how precious and perhaps nebulous life actually is. But it wasn't too long when the smiling Professor and his wife made an appearance and we quickly whisked them off to our house so that they could freshen up. I was still in disbelief that the Professor wanted to stay at our humble house as opposed to a luxury hotel, but was grateful nonetheless. The funny side of his visit was that we had never actually toured our own city, as Johannesburg is not exactly a tourist destination, but rather a large transit hub for idyllic African destinations. Anyway we obliged by planning as best we could by taking the Professor and his wife Doris to Lillieslief Farm where Nelson Mandela went into hiding, Lesedi Village for a quick African experience including eating 'delicious' mopani worms and a cable car ride up the Magaliesberg Mountain. Charlene as per usual had compiled a notebook with many questions with which to interrogate the professor. She asked her questions while I drove them to Lillieslief Farm and Professor Walz appeased her troubled mind with sensible answers. We took Calvin and Caleb out of school for their last day of touring and it also provided an opportunity for Prof. Walz to connect with Calvin, something that I was extremely grateful for. Our kind visitors had also spoilt both boys by giving Caleb a gigantic tub of sweets and Calvin got a much fancied Bayern-Munich shirt. The Professor and his gentle wife were a much needed panacea for us all and we soon bid them farewell on the next leg of their African Safari, for which they almost missed their flight.

We thereafter prepared for Calvin's treatment, but some of what Prof. Walz had shared with us regarding Calvin's surgery in Germany still echoed in my mind. He said that routinely they have to remove tumours that touch one or even two critical organs, but in Calvin's case it was five and the margin for error was usually not more than a millimetre. This amazing feat made me wonder as to the extent of what had been achieved with Calvin and I will remain forever grateful to these talented individuals.

Nuclear Medicine
It was 10 October 2014 and Calvin was admitted to the Donald Gordon Clinic. His room was on the furthest corner of the hospital festooned with radioactive warning signs. The room being on the top floor had a good view over the Johannesburg tree-line, but it still represented a three day prison sentence. A quick explanation was given regarding the dangers of radiation and the precautions to be followed. Thereafter, the radiation oncologist gave Calvin a truly disgusting mixture of iodine and milk to drink as protection for his thyroid gland. It so happens that the thyroid gland has a low threshold in resisting radiation and the risk of damage was a possibility. A drip stand arrived with an aluminium encased infusion that was condensing on the outside. Calvin's arm was prepared for the lethal infusion and soon the radioactive fluid was traveling through his veins. Calvin was henceforth not

allowed to receive visitors and all that was allowed were short periods of 10 minutes per person. As the day progressed so the allocated time was increased and soon it was possible to visit for 20 minutes at a time. As parents we had to be seated outside the door which led to some frustration, but it was necessary. Calvin received all his meals in disposable utensils, but this information did not filter down well to staff, resulting in perfectly good crockery being needlessly thrown away. The support that Calvin got from friends, teachers and family was amazing, and everyone showered him with attention and gifts. Three days later Calvin was back home none the worse for wear, however we knew that the after effects were yet to come.

Radiation is a double edged sword, effective in the treatment of various cancers but debilitating for specific sites in the body. Of concern to us was Calvin's white blood cell count and his thyroid function. These values correlated with the treatment received and we worked hard to reverse these effects. Despite this Calvin once again managed to end the year off on a high note by doing well in his final school results. Charlene had also started to plan a skiing trip that she long desired and arranged with our friends Tanja and Joerg to go to Austria on the 27 December 2014. However, as it would be our first skiing trip we would need to receive lessons at home and then in Austria. This new challenge refocused our minds. We practiced on a carpet slope in the late evenings of early December and had many fun moments, out of the family Calvin was definitely struggling the most, but he persevered even despite some worrying nose bleeds.

Calvin's Emotional Rollercoaster
Tragedy soon struck during this period and it would be Calvin's first real experience of death. His much loved dog Odie and companion for 10 years started to have seizures. I took her to the vet on a late Saturday evening thunderstorm as she had collapsed on the floor vomiting. The vet took her in and promised that he would try his best for her. That would be the last time

that I would see Odie. By Monday morning the vet said that she had made a remarkable recovery and we could collect her the next day. Unfortunately she never made that day as a seizure had eventually claimed her life. I received the news from Charlene at work and wondered how Calvin would cope with the loss. When I arrived home later that evening I could see that he was struggling through his emotions. Charlene had lit a candle next to a photograph of Odie, which made the atmosphere more sombre. We eventually sat down for supper and Calvin unexpectedly asked to say grace, and his sobbing prayer went something like this, "Dear God, thank you for letting me share Odie's life, she was the best dog a boy could have. Please look after her until the day that I can see her again. Amen." Well that was me pretty much finished, my emotions got the better of me and I darted from the table with tears streaming down my face. It was not the fact that Odie had passed that turned me into a pile of mush, but rather the sincerity in which Calvin made his solemn prayer. Through his prayer he'd had accepted both his mortality and afterlife together with his companion Odie, and it was all too much and too close to the 'bone' for me to handle.

That December turned into an emotional roller coaster, with Calvin seemingly working through his emotions and then regressing to a point in the evenings where he had to be calmed down by Charlene. By the time we left for our ski trip in Austria I had thought that the worst was behind Calvin. After an incredibly long flight we arrived in Munich airport just in time to catch a heavy snowfall, the excitement on the kids' faces was evident as we crossed the Austrian border on our way to Ellmau. The little town of Ellmau was picture perfect and better than what we had all imagined. That first evening Calvin had a complete 'meltdown' just before bedtime. He cried uncontrollably for his dog and Charlene was once again on hand to help him through his crisis. The end result was that I was banished to the sleeper couch with Caleb, but I was happy to oblige so long as Calvin was able to work through his emotions. During the day it was an altogether different play of events as he was having great fun on the slopes with his friend Florian and enjoyed the phenomenal food on offer at the hotel. Our friends are very accomplished skiers as they were brought up in the area and after our three days of training on the baby slopes they decided to accompany us to the proper mountain slopes. Once on top of the mountains our knees started to feel extremely wobbly and goodness only knows how we came down in one piece. However, both the boys progressed very quickly and in no time Caleb was following Tanja down the red slopes, while Calvin followed Joerg and Florian by skiing the more adventurous slopes including a few tricky black rated slopes. At the end of the holiday it was Calvin that had progressed way beyond expectation, a far cry from his struggles on the carpeted slopes of Johannesburg. Also with much effort from Charlene he had worked through his emotional baggage and was ready to take on the New Year. To this day both boys still regard the ski-trip as one of their best holidays.

A New Year
2015 started literally with a bang on the slopes of Ellmau and it took us some time to get back into the swing of the Jozi rhythm. Both boys were back at school, however Caleb was evidently struggling at his primary school. This prompted us to search elsewhere for something that could be more supportive. Charlene decided on a few options which prompted us to trying out new schools in succession, including De La Salle the school he initially had left. After some discussion between ourselves, we decided that De La Salle was the best option, but we soon realised that Caleb was lagging at his previous school. As such much catch-up was required from our part. Thankfully, he worked hard to catch-up and soon became an enthusiastic contributor on the sports field, playing in the soccer, cricket and rugby A-sides while loving every minute of it.

Calvin was enjoying high school and this was the year that he would need to decide on his subjects for the remainder of his schooling. We had him variously assessed with writing or accounting within the business field seeming to be a good fit. By March he did his usual 24 hour urine test which came back with absolutely normal values and both his thyroid function and white blood cell count was normal. However, Charlene was still battling the complexities of the paediatric oncology department, while Calvin had to endure many hours in an oncology room full of very sick children at various stages of predominantly chemo treatment. If anything these experiences made us all appreciate what we had, if you ever want to see real heroes just visit any paediatric oncology unit and you will come across heroic parents and their very determined children. Eventually August materialised and the all-important MRI scans were waiting for Calvin to verify the extent of the MIBG treatment performed the previous year. The scans happily revealed that the tumours had been reduced and the final diagnosis read as, "stable disease". Although we were happy with the results we still knew that he had the tumours in place and the prospect of them growing again was real, when this would happen was anyone's guess. However, Calvin felt great and was motivated to eat well and exercise. 2015 was his benchmark year, he dutifully pumped iron, ate his greens and avoided junk food, especially anything containing sugar. As the effects of the primary tumour had halted his club soccer, he was left with unresolved 'business'. He joined his old club after a two year absence, together with his younger brother. Unfortunately, his age group had changed significantly and the coaches were different and he never found his feet there. However, he joined a much faster form of 5-a-side soccer and played for his school, enjoying his beloved soccer one more time.

The 'Beast' Strikes Again
The seasons changed quickly and soon we were into our summer in October. I received a call one night from my sister Suzana in the UK and what she told me sent a shiver down my spine. She described how she was brushing her hair when she felt an un-

usual lump on her neck, she seemed not to be too concerned as she thought it could be a result of some dental work. My mind quickly raced at the mention of this, during our ordeal with Calvin I recalled seeing what was termed a 'glomus tumour' on a lady's neck and I knew that there could be some connection to our familial genetic link. Trying not to alarm her I suggested that she get to see a specialist right away so as to find out what the lump could be, but critically she would need to disclose to whomever she saw the occurrence of the gene in our bloodline. She evidently stumbled around the NHS system for some time before eventually getting the break she desired and saw the physicians at the Royal Free Hospital in London. The diagnosis was swift and it was confirmed that she did indeed have a glomus tumour that required surgical removal. In her case thankfully the tumour was still manageable and was not producing catecholamine, however there was a risk of nerve injury through the surgical procedure as the neck is a complex passageway. Suzana also half apologetically told me how sorry she was for not listening to my earlier recommendation to get a blood test, but that was in the past and there was nothing she could do other than tackle the matter on hand, and tackle she did. By February 2016 Suzana's own 'D-day' had arrived and her tumour was successfully removed, her recovery was swift with the loving support of her husband and children. The final obstacle to her ordeal was the dreaded genetic test that her children had to undergo as theoretically they had a 50% chance of having the gene. To speed up the process the genetic counsellor in London utilised our genetic data generated in Germany with permission granted by ourselves and Prof. Neumann. Unsurprisingly the genetic findings correlated with the SDHB mutation we had, but thankfully like our Caleb the mutation was not present in both her children.

Visiting Family And Tracing Our Heritage
By March 2016 Calvin once again completed his scheduled 24 hour urine test and all values as expected were normal. The first

half of 2016 went by quickly while I made plans for a family mid-year holiday in the UK and Portugal. The idea was that I would rather travel than have a party for my 50th birthday celebration. The trip would give me the opportunity to visit my sister Suzana and her family since I had not seen her post-surgery, it would also provide our boys with their first impressions of Portugal and a glimpse of their ancestral heritage. The boys completed their 2nd term of the year and both their school results were encouraging. In early August during their winter break we flew over to the UK. I had planned to stay four days with my sister and we arrived in the middle of her house renovations. From the word 'go' our boys and their cousins got on with each other as if the time that they had lost contact never existed. Caleb was in his usual element, acting like the clown that he is, while his cousins and brother fell all over themselves with laughter. We reconnected and time flew by almost too quickly. I was glad to see that my sister and her family were doing well. The next leg of our trip was Portugal, we arrived at the coastal town of Nazare in the middle of a blistering hot summer - luckily the sea breeze tempered the heatwave. We spent four balmy days with many funny moments in between, including Charlene's front crown breaking on a piece of marshmallow, an event that she would rather forget, but one that the boys continually recall.

After the break at the sea we headed 90 km inland to the mountainous region around Serta. The plan was to visit my father's inherited properties in a little village called Bravo where he was born and to visit two of his sisters and their families. In my wildest dreams I don't think I had ever imagined the boys retracing some of their grandfather's early footsteps, yet there they were clambering up every nook and cranny of the abandoned property. I eventually did see my aunts and we spoke about the diseases that the family had succumbed to. My father's only brother Caeser, the youngest in his family died in his thirties, leaving a wife and two young children. From accounts that I have heard over the years he seemed to have suffered from depression and anxiety. Coming from a small village in Portugal meant that the only way to cope with these conditions was through alcoholism. Eventually one day he could cope no more and took an agricultural poison to end his misery. By the time he arrived at hospital he was sober and remorseful, but it was all too late for him. My father's sister Belmira who Charlene once got to meet on an earlier trip was a very industrious person. She looked after her in-laws, her son and her husband, all the time while holding a job down as a cleaner for the local bank and selling baked goods at the local market. In late 2008 she was diagnosed with a tumour to the brain and she chose not to fight the disease, she took her own life at home. Subsequently her family fell apart, her in-laws passed away soon after that while her husband disappeared into alcoholism. In 1988 my otherwise healthy grandfather Rufino complained of pain in his stomach, he passed away after a short illness. The explanation from the village doctor was that he had some kind of cancer, again living in such a remote location meant having access only to the most basic medical services. In all three accounts is evidence of the genetic mutation, the anxiety and depression suffered by my young uncle is a common symptom of a catecholamine producing tumour. My aunt's brain tumour is a metastasis usually as a result of an undetected glomus tumour in female SDHB genetic carriers. My grandfather's extreme stomach pain is a symptom that Calvin also suffered from in 2010, an overproduction of catecholamine paralyses the smooth intestinal muscles making peristalsis painful. But in all three cases they had survived untreated well into adulthood, but the evidence although anecdotal was unmistakable.

We eventually wrapped-up our Portugal holiday on the sunny banks of the Tagus River at the very point where the Portuguese ships had long ago left for India via the African continent. Luckily for us our trip back to South Africa was quick and scurvy free.

Facing Our Worst Fear Again
Once we had arrived back home we focused on the task at hand

which was Calvin's annual scan. For some reason we had blocked this aspect out during our holiday, but we had increasingly become aware of Calvin's backache. After the scans were done Charlene met with Dr. Segal who by now was entrusted with Calvin's medical management, this after the frustration at the paediatric oncology unit. Our dealings with Dr. Segal over the years since he had first correctly diagnosed Calvin had grown into a mutually trustful relationship. The news from the scan report was rather confusing, the T12 tumour had shrunk a little more, while the sacral tumour had grown somewhat. The findings of the scan indicated the results were in keeping with "stable disease", however Dr. Segal was not happy with the increased vascularization evident on both lesions. He therefore asked that we have the scans seen to by his colleague Dr. Lohlun a radiologist oncologist for further assessment. A new wave of anxiety and worry washed over us and it felt like we had gone back to our initial pain of 2013. Charlene met with Dr. Lohlun who immediately assessed the situation and started email conversations with Prof. Neumann, she would be the only South African physician to do this. It was decided that to correctly assess the situation Calvin had to do a PET-CT scan. This scan could only be done at the Steve Biko Academic Hospital in Pretoria and the appointment was scheduled for early October 2016. Simultaneously I had started to read as many medical journals related to the subject that I could get my hands on. I spent many a late night absorbing as much as I could, making detailed notes as I went. My understanding of research developed through my work as an academic helped me to sift through what was pertinent and what was not. I would sometimes go to bed unable to sleep as my brain would be processing what I had read and in the morning I could not wait to discuss my findings with Charlene. I actually wondered if she thought that I was delusional when discussing alternative treatments, however she was also intent on listening and assessing what I had to say. Embolization and ablation were treatment options I had not yet heard of, but slowly that mystique unravelled. Calvin had also by this time became more pragmatic and despite having to study for his imminent exams still asked me to document everything that I had read into a file so that he could also read up later. Being a little older and wiser he understood the value of knowledge regarding his condition.

The day soon arrived for me and Calvin to take the trip to Pretoria, we landed up behind a long row of buses with the word "Star" emblazoned on the sides. It so happened that one ablation system that I had been reading about the previous night was trademarked as "Star", it seemed as if the message was clear. The Steve Biko Academic Hospital is an imposing structure, while the queue of cars, taxis and people was beyond belief. Once inside we made our way to the sixth floor where the Department of Nuclear Medicine was situated. The staff were extremely helpful and it was not long before Calvin was enduring a three hour long scanning procedure in an extremely cold, air-conditioned room. Once finished they handed me the discs and I raced back to Johannesburg to DHL courier to our friendly professors in Germany. In the meantime one article pricked my attention, it was an article discussing "malignant endocrine tumours" written by Professor Eric Baudin from the Gustave Roussy Institute for Cancer Treatment in Paris. It happened to be the most comprehensive article on the subject and it included a wide range of possible treatments for what Calvin had. I immediately sent an email to thank the Professor for his insightful article and enquired about the treatments that he detailed. At this point I had written already to a number of American doctors who had never responded, so I was extremely surprised when on the next day I received a response. In the email he described the "non-invasive" treatments to be the best options taken before opting for more systemic treatments. He also asked that I read up on a further article written by his colleague Dr. Frederic Deschamps, an interventional radiologist who specialised in cryotherapy (cryogenic-ablation) and cementoplasty. In other words tumours located in bone structure are frozen through a steel cannula inserted through the back and through the same cannula plastic cement would be delivered to fill the resultant cavity. This response was a real breakthrough in my search for an answer, but I stalled on the idea while I waited for the scan results and did further research.

Making Hard Decisions

The PET scan results eventually came and thankfully confirmed what we already knew. I had earlier intercepted one of the emails between Prof. Neumann and Dr. Lohlun in which the kind Professor intimated that he was hoping the PET scan would not reveal further issues. It was clear that Calvin still had the tumours that were always there at diagnosis, essentially the good news was that no new tumours had developed since diagnosis. Late one afternoon we met with Dr. Lohlun together with Calvin to discuss the way forward. Dr. Lohlun described through the use of the PET scans the precarious position of both tumours, for the first time we were given pictorial evidence and for us as parents it was an even more uncomfortable realisation. In her opinion the best treatment would be through stereotactic radiation, the treatment as I had previously read about was an effective option to stop tumour proliferation, but with a considerable list of long-term sideeffects. And so Dr. Lohlun best explained the process and then the effects, these ranged from stunted bone growth, secondary cancer, infertility, skin, bladder, nerve and spinal cord damage possibly leading to paralysis. On the flip side if the 'watch-and-wait' approach was utilised the long-term threat of bone collapse and paralysis was real, if there was a window for treatment opportunity it would be now. The treatment date was duly formalised. But before we left the doctor handed us a brochure in case we wanted to proceed with sperm collection, a matter than we found rather difficult to discuss with Calvin at such an early age.

Back at home we asked Calvin if in fact he wanted to have children some day and he matter-of-factly said "yes, I would like that". It was once more a point of mixed emotions as we were happy that he felt so clear about this, but sad at the same time for the ordeal he would have to endure to make this a possibility. In a very short space of time he was already making adult decisions. However, we remained extremely unhappy with the treatment option and we referred the matter to our German doctors. The response again was not what we expected as they agreed with our South African doctors that stereotactic radiation was the best route for treatment. Dr. Neumann highlighted the fact that the experience of the treatment in Germany was far superior to that of South Africa, however we knew if we elected to go to Germany we would not have medical aid cover as the treatment was available locally. We further prodded the German doctors on the possibility of alternative treatments, in specific ablation and cementoplasty. The response on this was muted and difficult to comprehend, but after much research I found that the process was not readily available in Germany, as in many other countries. I pressed Prof. Baudin from the Gustave Roussy Institute to get me into contact with Dr. Deschamps to which he obliged. Dr. Deschamps came back to me and said that their unit had great success in treating such tumours, however he would need to inspect the actual scans to assess whether Calvin would make an apt candidate for the treatment. That same day I arranged with the Pretoria based hospital to collect additional PET scans and rushed headlong down the highway with an energy that I cannot describe. En route I collected some chocolate to thank the staff at the hospital for organising this for me and proceeded to dispatch the scans to France.

While I was busy with the French option, Charlene through her Canadian friend Sarah got into contact with the Children's Hospital of Pennsylvania State (CHOPS). And, as per my previous experience with the American medical system we found communication extremely difficult. Even before we could speak to a doctor we had many documents to complete and had to pass through various levels of clearance before we had access to a doctor's opinion. We eventually got word that they would perform open surgery together with radiation treatment, this meant long term hospitalisation and an extremely long process of recovery.

Similarly another friend of a friend who had previous experience of cancer treatment in India sent our documents for an opinion. The Indian doctors suggested CyberKnife (another form of stereotactic radiation) paired with a course of systemic chemotherapy, he would be hospitalised for two weeks for a staggering amount of money. Further through my sister's contacts in the UK I found out that a unit was being made ready for the end of 2017 that offered minimally invasive treatments such as ablation and cementoplasty, however these would be managed by a physician from Strasbourg University in France, Dr. Afshin Gangi. I did some homework on this unit and the doctor and it offered us a second option if our Paris venture proved unsuccessful.

Waiting For The Green Light
An agonising week passed with no response from Dr. Deschamps and just as I started to despair a short email appeared to say that he was on a short holiday but that his assistant had received the scans and that he would give me feedback by Monday. I could breathe again but had to endure a weekend before his answer came back. Monday came and I was continually scanning my emails, while Charlene called to see if I had heard anything, her expectancy was also gradually mounting. I eventually drove home from work with still no news and as I parked my car in the garage my cell phone indicated that an email had just arrived. With a thumping heart I scanned my inbox and found what I was looking for. The email was succinct, Dr. Deschamps would be able to fully treat the T12 vertebrae - however the sacral bone was too risky. It was a bittersweet moment and very difficult for Charlene to accept as she hoped for full treatment. I fired another quick email and asked what other options we had for the sacral lesion. The response was swift, they would embolize the sacral lesion, in other words cut-off the veins that provide nutrients to the tumour and employ the 'watch-and-wait' approach. Charlene still not happy with the response sent an email of her own and asked what the option was if embolization failed. The answer was stere-

otactic radiation. We sat and discussed our options at length and quickly agreed that the French option was best, even if it required that we be more patient with the progress on the sacral lesion.

I duly instructed Dr. Deschamps that we wanted to proceed and he advised that from there onwards his assistant would arrange everything we needed. We also started the process of informing our medical aid that we were going to cancel the treatment in South Africa for the treatment in France. This required much paperwork, something we had got accustomed to. Soon after I received the quotation for the treatment and after a quick calculation found that it came close to $5000, could they have made a mistake? I quickly sent a query through to the assistant if the amount included treatment. The answer was simple "the amount includes the treatment". Not long after submitting the documentation to medical aid I too received the query whether the amount was correct. The email transcript between myself and the assistant was suffice to support the claim. It was very clear that as South Africans we have grown accustomed to the ever ballooning medical costs. From our previous experiences dealing with European countries we have noticed that their costs are remarkably realistic and the emphasis is on complete service. Our medical aid also required that we provide ample medical proof on the treatment that Calvin was to receive, this was not a problem as the French doctors were well published in the latest medical journals and their work was cited by other medical authors. Finding information on doctors based in Europe always seems easier than finding information on our South African doctors. On both occasions that we had procedures done in Europe we knew how the process happened and we were able to see the actual doctors working in their high-tech operating rooms. By the time we arrived in Europe we knew what the doctors looked like, how they were able to speak in English and what their facilities looked like.

Unfortunately the medical aid approval process took way too long and on top of this the French hospital would only confirm a treatment date once the payment was received. We dearly hoped to be able to make the journey to France before the end of November or latest early December, however we were placed in an uncomfortable position unable to do anything. Eventually by the second week waiting for an answer from medical aid we decided that irrespective if medical aid approved, we were going ahead and duly made the payment ourselves. Two days later we received the confirmation from the French hospital, our first appointment in Paris was to be on the 19 December and the treatment was set for the 20 December. The dates were a little on the late side of December but we were only too happy to oblige. A week later our medical aid eventually confirmed that they would cover 80% of the treatment costs. Thankfully we had gone ahead, had we waited for approval we would probably only have the treatment date in January, possibly jeopardising the start of Grade 11 for Calvin.

A Mother's Anguish
The travel and accommodation arrangements were the next issue to tackle. We had already in our minds and in discussion put out various options. December just happens to be a very tricky part of the year as our retail business is usually managed by Charlene and myself and it can get rather busy with Christmas sales. Then there was also Caleb who would be on his school holiday, who would look after him, while we were away? My proposal was that one of us would accompany Calvin and as the treatment was quick there would be no need to overdo things. Charlene on the other hand felt as the mother that she would like to be there. However, she did not want to travel alone with Calvin and in her own words said that she was "a nervous traveller who would more than likely stress Calvin out even more". Another option was that we all go as a family, however this was not to be a holiday and I could not imagine Caleb sitting still in and around hospital while Calvin received his treatment. I had also received a further instruction from the hospital, they wanted Calvin in Paris

at least 48 hours before and after his treatment. Charlene made a pact with me and said that she would discuss the dilemma of whether she should go or not with her friend Jane who happens to be a medical doctor with much experience. Eventually Charlene relented and said that her heart was broken, but that she knew I could handle the situation better and that it would be a further complication for her to go along since her travel documentation required a visa application. She finally said "Victor I give you my blessing to take Calvin to Paris". The best response I could muster was "don't worry we will be back before you know it". But this was not the end of this dilemma. And so I duly booked everything according to the hospital's request, we were to leave on the 14 December and return on the 23 December, arriving in time for Christmas Eve.

In all this time Calvin completed his exams and got involved in the matric dance committee together with Charlene. He was elected as the master of ceremonies for the event and had to arrange various fund raising activities in preparation for the matric dance. He also focused on his health being very conscious with what he was eating and stepped up his exercise in preparation for his treatment. He was going to be in the best shape possible so that he would be able to recover quickly. He read as much as he could on the treatment and watched through hospital videos Dr. Dechamps performing the treatment on various patients. Charlene had also got in touch with Dr. Craig Nossel CEO for Discovery Vitality and someone who has been very close to Calvin since his soccer playing days. Craig had always lended a helping hand in anything we did through our medical aid and this time it was no different. Since we were to go to Paris his suggestion was that Calvin go to Disneyland on the weekend before his treatment, he even offered to pay for this himself. It was a very kind gesture, but one that I was not comfortable in accepting, particularly since our sole objective was to have Calvin treated. Closer to our departure time Charlene ran into Craig and what he had to say put a 'spanner' in Charlene's head. He simply asked Charlene what was stopping her from going along to Paris. Soon after, Charlene came at me with, 'guns-blazing', she was coming along and that was her sole wish. I could not say anything else other than I would start the visa application process for her with the French Consulate. The next day I called her to confirm her interview appointment at the French Consulate, but her head was in turmoil, she abruptly said "I cannot think now, give me an hour to decide". I gave her the space she needed and she called me later in a subdued tone, "I guess I will just have to put on my big-girl panties and trust you on this". There was nothing more I could say or do on this issue other than to let it all be.

Meet You At Notre Dame

During the days before leaving Charlene spoke to her friend Ines who mentioned the prospect of contacting a mutual friend from our varsity days who lived in Paris. Within that same day Liz who we had long ago lost contact with called our home and enquired about Calvin and our Paris trip. As Charlene spoke to Liz on the phone I sensed that they connected as if the years passed had hardly changed. Liz started to make all sorts of arrangements with Charlene and soon she was sending me emails with various propositions. Quite funnily we made a date to meet one another that I will never forget, we would meet on Saturday at "15:00 in front of the Notre Dame Cathedral". Charlene also insisted contrary to my thinking that she would pay for Calvin to go to Disneyland as part of his Christmas gift and so we scheduled the Friday for this purpose. Since Friday and Saturday were already accounted for I suggested to Calvin that Sunday we would reserve for anything that he wanted to see or do in Paris. However, I knew that Calvin would be worn out by long-haul travel on top of having a full itinerary. His backache as result of the tumours had increasingly become more prominent, so this was an issue to be taken into account. I was also at that time running out of ideas for a Christmas gift for Charlene, however Caleb quickly came to the rescue with a special artwork that he had made at school. In his artwork pack was a collage made out of coffee beans and matches of the Eiffel Tower. I had his collage specially framed and we decided on an appropriate title that read, "tower of hope". Calvin's school friends had also made a video to wish him well while he was in hospital and his soccer team gave him a touching send-off. We were all primed to go and I just wanted to get to Paris fast and be back in time for Christmas.

Late on the afternoon of the 14 December my father dutifully collected us from home. The goodbye was rather heart-wrenching as Charlene could not control her emotions and as a result got Calvin in a teary state. Calvin soon composed himself as we made our way through the heavy traffic in the sweltering summer heat. After saying our goodbyes to my parents we headed through to the airport terminal and I indulged Calvin in a little retail therapy. I was only too happy to watch him trying out clothes and laughing at some of his more extravagant choices. In the back of my mind I knew that as much as possible I would need to divert his attention to other things other than the 'treatment' and having fun was going to be a big part of this divergence. Our flight on the big Airbus A380 was uneventful other than being extremely bumpy for most of the way. As we made our way into a wintery early morning Paris we quickly started to pick up visible landmarks like the Seine River and the Eiffel Tower beaming up a searchlight in our direction. We duly landed at 5:00 in the morning and once disembarked we proceeded through the various stages of the cavernous Charles de Gaulle Airport. Standing in long queues my ears soon became engulfed in the French language while I strained myself to make out what people were saying to one another. I was now truly isolated in a strange French world and would have my work cut out to get around my language disability. Once the formalities were done we headed to collect our luggage and then on to our pre-arranged shuttle, or so I thought. The waiting area at this time of the morning was not too busy and we walked through the exit chute looking out for my name. It was evident that not many people were being collected as there were only about seven names on display when we eventually walked through the line-up of boards. I was a little perplexed as I had meticulously arranged our collection, maybe our driver was still to arrive as it was rather early in the morning. We seated ourselves in the waiting area adjacent to the arrivals gate in hope of picking up our waylaid driver. After 30 minutes I gave up on the idea and went straight to the information desk to see if they could call the shuttle service, and they kindly called the number with no answer. But, then the lady at the desk informed me that there was a problem in Paris, the Uber drivers had blocked the roads around the airport in a protest against their unfair employment conditions. The only options to get out was to queue for the few taxis that were getting through or to take the train to the central Metro station, from there a tube ride to Villejuif and then a tricky bus ride to the apartment with all our luggage. We were both extremely tired and so we decided to wait in the bitter morning cold in the queue for the taxi. Our 20 minute wait felt like an eternity in the frozen morning air but eventually we were heading out of the airport, but as soon as we turned the corner away from the terminal building we ran into heavy traffic. It took us a further agonising hour to leave the airport precinct, all the while Calvin was happily dozing away on the back seat. Not too long after this point did we start to notice police activity and what seemed to be Uber cars stranded all over the road. We further observed more police kitted out from head to toe in riot gear, with eggs and flour strewn all over the road. At the end of the congestion we noted about 10 prison vans crammed with the objecting Uber drivers. I was relieved to have cleared the airport congestion and our driver propelled his car into 'hyper-drive' hurtling headlong towards our destination, but once again we ran into another problem, early morning Paris rush hour! Eventually we arrived over 2 hours later in Villejuif and immediately I could pick up the landmarks that I had mentally plotted from doing 'walk-throughs' on Google maps. Our driver following his GPS missed the turn off to our apartment and I had to bay for his attention to stop immediately lest we incur further unnecessary cost. Calvin looked at me surprised that I knew where we were, but I had already seen the Gustav Roussy Hospital in the background to know exactly where we were. The taxi bill was astronomical and I swallowed hard when I handed over the 102 Euros, but at least we had arrived at our destination.

Finding Our Parisian Feet
The apartment block was at the furthest periphery of the hospital complex right next to their extensive parking area. We slowly made our way with our luggage and entered the apartment reception area and were welcomed by the person on duty. After filling out the required forms we headed straight to our room and by now the coffee I had at the airport was expanding my bladder incrementally, I fumbled around with the key card and eventually the door swung wide open and to our absolute shock the bed was un-made and there was more evidence that we had gate-crashed someone else's room. I had visions of a similar incident in Paris many years back with Charlene, when we found a hotel staff member sleeping in our room. In disbelief we proceeded back to reception to complain and were quickly assigned another room. After packing our bags away we both crashed into bed to sleep our jet lag and morning's ordeal off. It must have easily been the best sleep we both had in a while as we slept sweetly for over four hours. Feeling restored we next focused on trying to FaceTime Charlene, this was going to be our first experience using this communication technology and we soon found out that using it as a standard telephone was infinitely better than trying to see each other and speak. In our conversation Charlene asked what our view was like of Paris, and we opened our curtains up to a very busy road with a bus stop opposite an abandoned yard whose gate was covered in graffiti and a gaudy advertising board facing our room. I chuckled to myself as the thought of being in magical Paris for Charlene was completely unlike the reality that I faced.

After our lengthy conversation we readied ourselves for the mission of the day. We first needed to go to the hospital to notify the doctors that we had arrived and were on track for our Monday appointment. The next most pressing matter was getting our groceries for the days ahead. Outside light was fading and by now the wintery sun was doing a poor job of heating up the earth so we needed to get out fast lest we wanted to walk around a strange town in the dark. We made the 800 metres to the hospital in no time while passing various hospital laboratories and buildings along the way. The hospital's sculptural water tanks flanked our left and I could not help to notice that the mortuary was in the middle of our route. Once we swung right and away from the water tanks the imposing entrance to the Gustave Roussy Cancer Hospital was straight ahead of us, looking exactly like the internet images that I had previously explored. We entered the enormous reception area and stood in a short queue. With our patient documents in hand we notified the English speaking attendant that we had arrived in time for our Monday appointments, and in return he gestured to us that they had taken note of this. With this little formality behind us we made way to where I knew shops to be located. Since I do enjoy different eating experiences I was looking forward to buying some local produce for our table. En route we found two bakeries and a supermarket with an English name - Leader Price. Top of our grocery list was baguettes, croissants, quiche, cheese and cold meat cuts. We were loaded like pack mules for our trip back to our room and to my surprise the bill was very fair, particularly for our depressed South African wallet. Calvin and I dined better that evening than what any Parisian restaurant could offer. He chatted excitedly about our day's adventures and the Disneyland excursion for the next day. Hospitals, doctors and procedures were furthest from both our minds that evening.

Searching For Disneyland

The next morning we hurriedly ate our breakfast while I studied the intended route to Disneyland. Once outside the bitingly cold air was unmistakable, this was winter and we had to adapt quickly. I noticed that fog had accumulated all around us, but at least it wasn't raining. The no.182 bus to the Paul Couterier tube station arrived on schedule while I readied our bus fare for payment. Now if you have never done this in a strange country with a different language what was about to happen can only be explained as fantastical. As I entered the bus I failed to pick up the sign that read "gratuit" and proceeded to shove my cash in the direction of the bus driver to which he mumbled something that vaguely felt like I was being rejected. Once the driver pointed at the "gratuit" sign I understood that he was not interested in taking my cash and I made my way to the back of the bus to where Calvin was sitting. As I was about to take my seat an elderly gentleman seated in front of Calvin abruptly explained that the air pollution levels in Paris were high and therefore to alleviate the problem all public transport was free. Then he asked "are you English?" to which I replied in an almost proud manner "no I am South African from Afric du Sud". Well it was priceless the expression on the gentleman's face, I almost thought that he might even get up and give us a hug. It turned out that he hailed from Tunisia and had just recently visited South Africa and in no time at all was showing me images on his mobile of his visit to Kruger National Park, Mandela Square, Cape Town and Robben Island. In his excited state he referred to me as his African brother from the South. Then suddenly his expression changed and he asked me what I was doing in Villejuif, to which I explained we were there because we had an appointment at the Gustave Roussy. Being a resident to Villejuif he knew full well what we were there for and his next question was straight as an arrow, "where is his cancer?" I gave him a succinct explanation and then he asked me to take his mobile number in case I had any problems, he lived around the corner from the hospital. Abdel Isaac was his name and for a man of considerable age he was very sharp. His next deduction once again was spot on when he said "now you visit Paris - Le Torre Eiffel?" To which I answered "no we are going to Disneyland". Without any prompting he offered to show us the way to where we could transfer to the train line leading to Disneyland, he did not want us to worry about what trains or stations to choose as he knew exactly where to take us. Again in his excited state he lost track of where the tube train was going and I being more geographically inclined suggested that we were going in the wrong direction, to which it only actually dawned on him about three stations later that indeed we were heading deep into Paris. With any further delay averted we hurriedly changed trains onto the direction of the correct train line. Eventually Abdel bade us good-bye at the intersection point and wished Calvin well for the treatment.

The train slowly rumbled out of central Paris and as we emerged out of the underground system I noted that the sky was perfectly clear, the fog had somehow lifted and the day held the promise of sunshine somewhat like a South African Highveld's winter's day. On the train ride I reflected on what had happened as I could not believe that in the middle of the chaos a Good Samaritan took charge of us to ensure our well-being in his city. He was an older Muslim gentleman who I would not have considered to be helpful. Our commonality being that we were from 'Africa', but in reality we were very different and somehow still the same. This event confirmed to me the concept of 'angels amongst us', in all our travels and ordeals it was people that always made the difference.

Visiting Disneyland for me was a surreal experience. In my wildest dreams I may have never considered a visit to this fabled institution, however I know all kids would relish an opportunity to be there. Since it was Calvin's gift from Charlene I pretty much stood back and let him enjoy the experience, for me it was special to see that he could revel in this small opportunity. Throughout our visit we would talk about Caleb and what he would have thought of the experience. It's funny how we walked around the park never once forgetting about Charlene and Caleb back home, it was as if they were right there next to us all the time. Our experiences were both funny and exhilarating, punctuated by the occasional shopping spree and enjoying some down time over a cappuccino. In my focus to ensure that Calvin's treatment ensued without a hitch I had just about forgotten about Christmas. Disneyland and Christmas are just about as inseparable concepts as you can get, it was unmistakable, Christmas had truly arrived. From the decorations, music, non-stop parades, *gluhwhein* and the biting cold, all played the role to finally bring the Christmas spirit to me. Everything went down smoothly until our ride in the haunted house broke down and we chilled-out by sharing some *biltong* (beef-jerky) while people ran around frantically to sort the problem out. Eventually after our *biltong* was finished we were asked to leave our seats and walk out of the haunted house, on our way out we had a good look at all their 'trade' secrets. As night time drew closer and the park got more congested we realised that in all our excitement we had forgotten that the shops were about to close and we had yet to buy Charlene and Caleb their gifts. In a flash we made our way to the store that we had earlier earmarked for our purchases and piled my backpack full of gifts which included a very realistic Star Wars light-sabre that kept buzzing on and off as I walked around the park. I had second thoughts on traveling with the light-sabre due to its length, but Calvin insisted that I take it, this decision would provide us with many funny moments as I travelled back to South Africa with it. By this time it was pitch dark and crowds of people thronged around the magical Disney castle, but all I wanted to do was to get out of the park as I was worried about finding our way back to the apartment on the public transport system. Calvin however begged me to stay as he felt that all the people were there to see something big. Eventually I relented and to my absolute surprise we stood there in amazement as a stunning fireworks display framed the fabled castle in exploding light, a fitting send-off to Calvin. Charlene's present to Calvin could not have been more perfect.

Back-Pain In The City Of Lights

After making our way back to the apartment late that night I was thankful that Calvin had not complained about the pain in his back, until we were on the train. The pain was starting to stymie any efforts that he had of enjoying himself, but at least it had held back all the way through our Disney experience. We eventually woke up late the next morning after our exhausting adventure the day before. After a good breakfast it was decided that we would leave later to make our way to Paris for our appointment with Liz and her family in the afternoon. We made our way back into Paris and by now I was more confident in getting around town. We got out of the nearest tube station to the Notre Dame Cathedral and had a good laugh at a 'self-cleaning' toilet. The afternoon was crisp and sunny while people milled about cafes while enjoying a cornucopia of heated beverages. We paused for a while listening to buskers playing on the bridge behind the imposing structure of the cathedral. As we made our way to the front of the cathedral a long snaking queue greeted us. Since we were early for our appointment we decided to join the queue with the other visitors. As we entered the cathedral my mind raced back to 2010 when Charlene and I had been in the very same place. Charlene at the time was particularly preoccupied by having left Calvin home battling a mystery ailment, she dutifully lit a special prayer candle for him. Now six years later here we were closing the prayer loop that Charlene had started. At the very same place Calvin lit his prayer candle, something that I will never forget as long as I live. The cathedral was also decorated for the Christmas period which added that special sparkle to our humble occasion.

Once outside again we decided to enjoy some coffee Parisian style at the nearest cafe and marvelled at the continued throng of people visiting the famous landmark. After warming ourselves up with coffee we returned to the front of the cathedral and waited for our friends. I stood there trying to imagine if after all these years I would still be able to recognise them or if they would recognise me. My question did not take long to be answered as we instantaneously recognised one another, yes we were all older but somehow we were still the same. It did feel good that we were not alone in this huge city, Liz was accompanied by her husband Michael and their daughter Gabriella and younger son David. As Liz had planned a rather busy night out in Paris we briskly made our way to the Latin Quarter for something to eat. Gabriella being Calvin's age connected right away with him, in fact I was surprised how their kids being brought up in France had quite pronounced South African accents. More impressive is that they mastered not only French and English, but also Liz's native language Portuguese and German that was being taught at school. We spent a relaxed afternoon together with Liz and Michael asking as many questions as they could about Calvin. Both remarked as to Calvin's exterior appearance, as was the case with many of our other friends - they would never have guessed that he had cancer. But then again Calvin was fortunate not to have ever undergone chemotherapy, as that treatment does produce all the hallmarks of a cancer sufferer.

After our meal Liz explained her plan for the rest of the evening. She was not going to rest until she had shown Calvin the 'city of lights' by night. Our first stop was the Louvre gallery but unfortunately we were a little late, but I explained to Calvin that even with a full day it would be virtually impossible to see everything. Nonetheless we made our way to the central entrance and we all touched the lower apex of the famous glass pyramid. After which Gabriella said her farewell as she was going to work that evening - she was au-pairing for a young family at the time. In the short time that I met Gabriella it became quickly apparent how mature and level headed she seemed, no doubt the loving upbringing that she enjoyed. We further milled around the shopping mall in wonder of all the fascinating merchandise. By the time we rendezvoused again with Liz and Michael, I noticed little David playing it up with mom, something not so different at our house. Eventually David was given the object of his immediate desire - a big luminous spinning top. He spent the rest of his way back to the car spinning the top and explaining the many ways to operate the fascinating toy. Having David's energy around made me miss Caleb terribly, but I had to console myself that this was not an ordinary trip.

Soon we were driving down the famous Champs Elysees and made our way to the illuminated Eiffel Tower. In the manic traffic Liz asked for me and Calvin to alight and to watch the tower. We stood there in the cold evening admiring the light adorned tower while taking numerous images. All of a sudden the tower's lights started to pulse in hyper-rhythm which made the already glittering landmark even brighter, we just stood there in awe, not quite believing that we were witnessing it. For the rest of the evening Liz hunted down many of the top landmarks and special amongst those was the Sacre Cour Cathedral on Mount Matre. It was my first time visiting this Cathedral on the hill overlooking the city and we both enjoyed the experience completely. The visit also made me appreciate the fervent faith that Liz and Michael displayed. Our final sight-seeing stop was the Galleries Lafayatte shopping complex with its street display windows crowded with onlookers. The famous Paris shop had as per usual gone all-out with Christmas decorations, something that I had never seen, but there I was munching on roasted chestnuts in the cold while observing the spectacle all for myself. As we made our way back to the car again I overheard Liz and David in a heated discussion about where to go and have late supper. He was hoping for KFC like all respectable 11 year olds and I think Liz wanted something more local. I couldn't resist but to lend my support to David's cause lest he behave like Caleb after not getting his way, Liz eventually relented and made her way to KFC to David's delight. I think it was way past midnight when Liz dropped us off in front of our apartment after refusing to leave us to find our own way back. David had long dropped off to sleep at the back of the car, but we said our goodbyes and Liz promised to visit Calvin in hospital. Unfortunately for all their kindness they still had a long way to get back to their home on the other side of Paris, but I could only offer Liz and Michael my humble appreciation for what they had done for myself and Calvin. We had in that time forgotten that we were far away from home.

Calvin's Last Run

The next morning we slept-in as Calvin needed to recoup some of his strength. It was Sunday and the last day that we had at our disposal for more sightseeing. Calvin wanted to do a boat trip and a visit to Napoleon's last resting place, the Hospital des Invalides. We made our way back through the now familiar Paris Metro and arrived at the embarkation point nearest the Notre Dame Cathedral. The ticket booth attendant asked for our identification documents and as we were travelling as European citizens I produced our Portuguese ID cards. I stood there momentarily watching the attendant's brow deepen as he examined the documents. The attendant eventually asked "you speak perfect English for a Portuguese", to which I replied "you are French, how can you tell the difference?". His knowledge of the language was picked-up over many years working as a ticket attendant in probably one of the busiest places on the planet, and he could tell an American apart from an Englishman, however my South African accent coupled with my Portuguese ID card had him confused. Eventually after a friendly chat he convinced himself that we were indeed a hybrid breed that spoke the best English he had ever heard or at least an English he could clearly understand. Soon we were relaxing inside the warm glass cocoon of the boat while taking in all the famous sites. Our seats faced to the back of the boat where a young girl and her selfie-stick had us truly entertained with her antics, it was freezing outside and it was a miracle that she could even muster a pout.

We visited the Eiffel Tower once again and then headed straight to the Hospital des Invalides. On our way we passed young Parisian men without shirts out in the cold park playing a game of soccer, we were impressed not for their ball skills but their ability to go shirtless in the middle of a freezing afternoon. After having gone through a very thorough security inspection at the entrance by deadly looking legionnaires we were allowed to enter the museum. Unfortunately, time was against us so we decided to head straight to the section that housed the exhibits of the Napoleonic era. The museum is truly impressive if not a tad overwhelming, but we were both entranced by what we saw and sadly after spending over two hours we had to make our way to the exit. Once outside the blast of the cold air took us a little by surprise but we managed a brisk walk in the dark to catch the boat back. Once we got near to the river I heard the unmistakable grumble of the boat on my left and realised that if we did not catch this boat it would be a long wait in the cold for the next boat. I turned to Calvin and asked "how are you for a run?" He looked at me and said "I'm fine, let's go!" With that we both shot-off into the dark desperately trying to stay ahead of the boat as it made its way to the next stopping point. The boat looked deceivingly slow and yet it was making distance on us, soon we realised that we were in a futile race, the boat was too fast. Running in thick winter clothing with a heavy backpack is something that I last did in my army days and I had no joyful memories of that time as I was puffing onwards. We had already covered a distance of about two kilometres when I noticed that to stop, the boat would need to slow down and manoeuvre itself into the disembark position. That's when I shouted to Calvin who was ahead of me to keep on running as we could still make it and indeed we did. We stood there waiting for the passengers to disembark blowing big steam clouds into the cold air, but glad that we had made it. We had run for about three kilometres and as I now recall that was going to be Calvin's last run in a long while. We were both grinning from ear to ear, happy to have warmed up and happy to be heading to a warm apartment. Once we had made it back to our apartment we headed straight to the nearest bakery to stock up on croissants for Calvin's breakfast. We called Charlene and Caleb back home and went to bed tired and content, but pensive about the next day.

Meeting Dr. Deschamps

Monday morning eventually dawned and we made our way to the hospital for our 9:00 appointment with Dr. Deschamps. The hospital building was a hive of activity and in the process we got lost somewhere inside its vast corridors. We eventually found our waiting room and waited while we observed the people around us. First thing that struck us was the age of the patients, they were all old and mostly men. Then we couldn't help notice that at every reception point was a young good looking girl, which made me wonder about the hospital's hiring strategy. When Dr. Deschamps made an appearance he went straight to an older couple and shook the gentleman's hand and they disappeared into his consulting room. Since we had already seen Dr. Deschamps doing operations online and presenting his findings at medical conferences we had no trouble in identifying him. Dr. Deschamps looked to be in his thirties and stood well over 6 feet. Like the other doctors at the Gustave Roussy he wore a distinct white overcoat. It was evident that the process of ablation in its various guises was popular amongst the elderly as it dealt with the debilitating pain of spinal conditions. We had observed various operations online where ablation was used to deal with problematic spinal nerves relieving patients of their pain. Eventually it was our turn and we walked into the consultation room. Dr. Deschamps greeted us and tentatively asked if we understood French, to which I replied, "Doctor, your English is infinitely better than our French could ever be". Dr. Deschamps in his thick French accent obliged us by first describing to Calvin how these tumours had developed and what his plan for restoration was going to entail. This was the moment that another spanner was flung into my internal workings. Firstly he changed our initial arrangements by saying that he would operate on Calvin on the Wednesday and not the Tuesday as Calvin was required to undergo some vital tests prior to the procedure. But he quickly turned and said that we were fine to still leave on the Friday as one day was more than enough to recover in hospital. His second point was probably even more disturbing, he suggested that as

Calvin was young and healthy enough they were going to attempt the full treatment of both tumours and not just partial treatment as previously discussed. I probably looked like a fool as I could not counter any of these new propositions, things were just moving too fast for me to even think. Dr. Deschamps then took out a piece of paper where through the use of drawings explained what he was going to do. What was interesting was that in order to treat the T12 vertebra the only access point was at an oblique angle through Calvin's side via the lung chamber. The left lung would be blown up out of the way of the cannula with CO_2 gas. As for the problematic sacral tumour the plan was to do cryoablation, but to reduce the freezing cycle and deliver cementoplasty under pressure into the affected cavity where the polymer's curing reaction would cause the opposite effect as it produced heat. In Dr. Deschamps opinion this was going to be the best chance he would have of a full recovery. Calvin's hospitalisation plan was that he be admitted to the hospital the next day in preparation for the procedure on the Wednesday and he was to be discharged on the following day.

After our appointment with Dr. Deschamps we made our way to see the oncologist who also turned out to be a very young doctor. Dr. Fresneau also spoke English and had an astonishing knowledge regarding pheochromocytomas. He did a few cursory tests on Calvin and asked him very pertinent questions. He then turned to me and said that in Calvin's case the fact that he had not developed any new tumours since his diagnoses and also that the spinal tumours had remained more or less the same size since detection was a very good sign going forward. He intimated that whatever he was doing that he keep that up, this obviously included the rigorous screening protocol that he had followed to date. From there we had an appointment with the chief anaesthetist and explained Calvin's bad episode coming out of anaesthesia in Germany. He took note of the issue and explained that there were a variety of methods in which they handled the problem, but essentially he would ensure that I would be on hand when Calvin transitioned back to consciousness after the operation. With all our appointments done we headed straight back to our apartment and took stock of our situation. So much had been discussed that I needed some breathing space to organise my thoughts and rearrange our schedule. My first thought was to inform Charlene of the changes as no doubt she would be preparing herself mentally for the procedure that was supposed to happen on the next day. I also knew that the school had arranged a church service to be held at more or less the time Calvin was being operated on. Plus the fact that the procedure had changed to what we as parents originally wanted, but possibly dreaded. So this was a rather tricky situation that I had found myself in.

"What do you mean both his tumours are getting the full treatment? Couldn't they have told us earlier about the changes? What will I tell all the people at the school?" Charlene like myself was thrust out into unknown territory, somewhere between a 'rock and a hard place'. It took a while to convince Charlene that we were on the right track and that I felt confident in Dr. Deschamps abilities to successfully treat Calvin. In essence Calvin was going to get the full treatment and to come out all that way to 'chicken-out' at the last minute by turning down this opportunity was not in Calvin's best interests. After reaching a consensus Charlene reminded me to show Calvin the video his friends at school had made before he left for France. After fumbling around on my iPad I eventually found the video clip and played it for Calvin. In the video all his school friends and teachers wished him well. It was touching to see how much they all loved him and he enjoyed every minute of it. He did not expect this gift at that time, especially after all the 'heavy' stuff done at the hospital that morning. For a brief moment I could see that he was transported back home where his heart was.

Another Hospital, Another Procedure

The next morning we took the bus to a shopping complex nearby, by the intriguing name of " Le Vache Noir" or the 'black cow', we were unsure if this name would fly back home though. Our plan was to shop for gifts for our family before returning home. In reality I just wanted Calvin to get some shopping therapy and I was ready to indulge him. Calvin tried on many outfits, some ridiculous others very Parisian, but he was having fun. He eventually chose for himself an outfit that he could travel back home with. However, the jeans that he chose in my opinion looked like they were ripped off a hobo. Once our shopping was done we headed back to the apartment for something to eat before eventually making our way back to the hospital. Calvin was assigned to a room at the furthest corner of the adolescent corridor in the paediatric wing. Because we were designated as 'African' we were to be quarantined and treated like we had the Bubonic plague, however this afforded Calvin the use of a private ward. Like in our German experience we were given very long cotton buds for all his orifices, however we saved nurses from explaining what to do, by now we were expert users. Outside the door a huge stand was placed with a warning sign and all the protective clothing that medical personnel required to have on when doing tests on Calvin. As this is an academic hospital all the tests were conducted by medical students, as such it became very amusing as group upon group of students came in and not only struggled to speak to us, but were squirming in badly fitting protective clothing. A few hours later once the tests confirmed that Calvin was not carrying Armageddon all the precautions were lifted, unless of course the staff grew tired of all the unnecessary protocol.

Later in the afternoon we met Dr. Marion, the internist Doctor, she luckily spoke English and had recently visited South Africa, unlike the students we had seen before her. She explained the procedure for the next day, Calvin was to avoid eating after supper and only have water if needed in the evening. He was required to be bathed in a special soap, have his operation gown on and be ready by 7:00 the next morning. With the formalities done we settled as best we could for the first night in hospital, being in the paediatric ward made us attuned to the noises of sick children and babies. We observed parents doing shift work between holding jobs and caring for their precious bundles, it was heart wrenching to see. On our side we noted that all the teenagers were bald due to the effects of chemo, however their mood seemed stoic and altogether a different approach was needed in their care. We also could not help but notice the overtly Christmas ambience of the ward, but how does one even contemplate Christmas in a place like this? Occasionally, ruptures of laughter would break out when a visiting clown arrived to cheer up the young ones, but soon all this died down and it was back to wails and beeping monitors. Calvin hardly touched his supper and settled down into an uncomfortable sleep, while I tried to master sleeping on the sleeper chair. I eventually solved my problem by starting to write the second part to our story. Funny how when I write I disappear into another world and it wasn't long when I too fell into an uncomfortable sleep.

D-Day 3

My phone alarm rudely woke me up just as I thought I had found the sweet spot for a comfortable snooze. I woke Calvin up and readied him for our 7:00 am rendezvous with destiny, in the process I recalled doing this a few years earlier in Germany. It somehow all felt familiar to me. Not a minute past seven and the hospital attendants appeared ready to take Calvin to the operating theatre. I followed Calvin's wheeled bed into the bowels of the enormous building, slowly making our way through various security entrances. Calvin's bed was parked alongside another patient while I was asked to change into theatre clothing, something that took me by surprise, but then I remembered the conversation that I had with the anaesthetist. From there Calvin was wheeled into the theatre and I was dumbstruck with what I saw. I truly felt that I was inside a spaceship, there was a hive of activity with medical personnel dressed top to toe in theatre garb, all focused on the task. Calvin was lifted onto a narrow stainless steel table on rollers directly opposite a CT scan machine. In an adjoining room behind a glass window I could see a collection of computer monitors with various personnel in attendance. All the monitors that I could see had Calvin's scans with a myriad of lines and target points, no doubt the prior planning done by Dr. Deschamps. I noted that Dr. Deschamps was conspicuous by his absence, but like all maestros the ground work needed to be carried out by the lower rung functionaries. In my view he would arrive, do his magic and quickly leave, but that was my naive interpretation. As Calvin lay on the operating table the anaesthetist arrived and connected a tube on the IV line already in place. At the same time she asked Calvin if he wanted to be a doctor, to which he mumbled something vaguely to do with business. But I appreciated her attempt to relax Calvin. I watched a white fluid travel into his body while I stroked his hair and re-assured him that all was going to be well. His eyes were moist and I sensed a certain connection between the two of us, it was an emotional moment for me to see him drift-off to another place - he was there physically, but his persona had gone.

The walk back to the paediatric ward was long and thoughtful. I tried hard not to think about anything in particular, but it was a futile task. As I walked into the room the cleaners were busy cleaning every nook and cranny, so I decided to take a walk down the passage. It was breakfast time and parents were sitting in the cafeteria trying their best to feed unwilling children, but they pressed on with patience. By the time I returned to the room the cleaners had gone and I resigned myself to wait the time out there. The room was eerily empty without Calvin. I again busied myself in the best way that I knew and that was to write. But the time in that room was excruciating if not uncomfortable and thankfully it ended sooner than I had anticipated. A nurse popped his head in and said "monsieur dos Santos s'il vous plait", I did not need a second invitation to move my butt. My heart was in my throat as I made my way to the operating station, but was again required to dress appropriately. I entered the recovery room and noticed that there were about 12 patients in various stages of consciousness, however I could not help but notice that only one of those patients was doing a lot of movement in bed. It was Calvin and he was at the head of the room with a huge television screen playing what seemed to be *The Avengers* at full blast. The first thing he asked me was to switch the offending TV off and then he turned and said, "this was nothing compared to Germany". I was ecstatic because he could move his legs and was not paralyzed. I asked Calvin how he felt and he seemed to be in good spirit, with no visible sign of trauma. Dr. Deschamps eventually made his way to us and recounted what they had done to Calvin. In his opinion their objectives were achieved and Calvin would be discharged the next day, which was good news to me. However in retrospect our next challenge was only about to begin.

Calvin was wheeled on his bed back to his room. He had endured a 2 hour procedure and 45 min post-operative observation in the recovery ward, in his mind he was ready to go home. But alas our day had just begun, the anaesthesia was still coursing through his body so pain was negligible, but he was now suffering from bouts of nausea. As much as he tried to control his nausea it kept on building until his sweaty, shivering body could no more and he threw up all over the bed. The ward nurses were quick to clean up and make him as comfortable as possible. This time they left a kidney shaped tray so that he had a dedicated vomit receptacle. But this option failed dismally when the next bout of nausea resulted in an almighty gush of liquid that all but missed the now useless kidney tray. The nurses once again cleaned up, but this time they said that if he vomited again they would require that he be moved to the chemo room. Calvin looked at me a little perplexed, but I explained that the chemo room was designed to accommodate sick patients prone to vomiting. That bit of information did the trick on Calvin as he stopped vomiting altogether for some time. He managed to get some sleep in the afternoon and woke up a while later to ask that I bath him so that he could get dressed into his pyjamas, up until that point he was still butt-naked. I had seen earlier that he had little strength in his legs and assumed it was still too early for the effects of the operation to have fully resolved. So this time I asked him to get to the edge of the bed while I disconnected the IV line. Once in position I asked him to stand and with that he fell into a heap at my feet like a sack of potatoes. It was both funny and worrying but eventually he walked the few steps to the bath while leaning heavily on me. I set about removing plasters that were stuck in uncomfortable places on his body, however these were plasters like no other that I had seen. I almost had to scald Calvin to just nudge them a little, but they left a nasty residue for some time to come. His operation scars were no bigger than pin-pricks, an amazing feat considering what he had endured. In the process of cleaning Calvin nausea once more set in, he was burning up and the perspiration trickled off him in sheets. He vomited once more but luckily he was sitting on a suspended chair slightly above the draining water, so avoided being bathed in his own vomit. Once bathed and tucked back into bed he felt a whole lot better, he even attempted to eat some yoghurt. We had a short chat with Charlene on the phone to reassure her that all was well and I headed back to the apartment to shower and get ready for the night in hospital with Calvin.

The Challenge Of A Hospital Recovery

Sleeping in hospitals is a skill that I do not excel in. Just the mere thought of sleeping another night gave me cold shivers. The worst part of the proposition was that I knew Calvin's pain was going to increase as the effects of the anaesthetic subsided, all this while we both struggled to find some sleep. I made up most of the early evening by either chatting to Calvin, writing or just looking out the window trying to relive some of the days moments. My thoughts went back to an earlier incident as Calvin was transitioning out of sedation. As he lay there half-conscious he started to talk in a low tone, "dad, who will look after me when I leave home?" It was a deep question and without reservation I said, "Calvin my boy, you will always be our son no matter how old you are and it means that we will always work hard to ensure your health no matter where in the world you are". I then asked "are you worried when you leave home to study?" To which he replied "yes, but I also know all this costs money and takes a lot of effort for you and mom to arrange". Calvin was realising that he was no longer a child, but a bigger child becoming a young adult and as such he needed some reassurance on his future care. It was also an admission of his own vulnerability and dependence on us as parents. I eventually just held his hand and said that he should not worry, especially now that he was supposed to recover from his operation. With that he turned over and went to sleep while I struggled to hold back my own tears.

The beeping IV monitor rang out while I was deep into some troubled sleep. Calvin had pinched the line shut in his sleep and the alarm was there to warn staff that his medication was not reaching his body. The door swiftly opened and the nurse readjusted the line once more. This event happened many times over as Calvin moved around in bed. Later in the early morning I could no longer sleep on the chair and I decided to lay my blankets on the floor. The change of posture gave me much relief and I slipped back to sleep only to be woken up again by the night nurse accidentally tripping on my floored body while she checked up on Calvin. Somewhere in the early morning Calvin also needed the toilet and this process required much shuffling around the room to avoid him falling on something hard. Thankfully the ward lights came on early as a signal that we had made the morning, I opened our curtain and saw the early Paris traffic snaking in the cold wet distance. Calvin lay sound asleep, the lights did little to disturb his sleep. I sat there contemplating his struggles with standing and walking, hoping for an improvement. My concern was that Calvin needed to be more mobile as we were leaving for home the next evening. But I banished my concerns and focused on what needed to be done on the day.

My task for the day was to speak to Charlene and run through what was going to happen in preparation of our imminent departure. I also needed to speak to Dr. Deschamps regarding my concerns for Calvin, including discharge and plans for his recovery at home and re-scanning. Lastly, I also needed to touch base with Liz as she was planning to visit Calvin that afternoon. On top of all this there was the matter of gifts that I had brought along to give to key staff, but unfortunately I did not have a gift for one of the young nurses who really tried hard with Calvin. I decided I would get a box of chocolates from the hospital shop. Now giving gifts in South Africa may seem very pedestrian or even the expectation, I was just about to transgress a cultural divide on top of losing things in translation. Eventually Dr. Dechamps made an appearance in the late morning. He seemed upbeat about the results of the treatments on Calvin and again reiterated what was achieved. He ensured me that Calvin would recover in time and that he would prescribe some pain medication to take with us. I thanked him for all his efforts and then gave him a Nelson Mandela notebook which he humbly accepted and wished Calvin well on his journey back home. With that he left the room, the discharge note he said would be signed by Dr. Marion the ward internist. A little later nurse Pauline made an appearance and I thanked her for looking after Calvin, especially since she did her best to communicate in English. I handed her the box of chocolates which unfortunately the lady at the shop misunderstood my requirement and went all out with extravagant wrapping. Nurse Pauline refused profusely to take the gift, but I convinced her it was only chocolates to which she eventually relented. I then took out my phone and gestured to her that I wanted a photo with her and Calvin. Well if I had ever muddled things up then this was a very good example of me not being able to 'read-between-the-lines'. Nurse Pauline immediately jumped back and said to me, "no, no, not allowed", while Calvin reading the whole situation leaned over to me and said "dad, she thinks you want her mobile number". That was enough for me to whip my phone back into my pocket and watch the young nurse awkwardly extract herself from our room. Needless to say we never saw her again, I could just imagine her saying to her colleagues how this older South African guy was so rude, that despite having a sick son he had no qualms in making uncomfortable advances on her. After that incident Calvin and I cracked up in laughter, but we needed the humour.

The End Of The Road...Or So I Thought

Dr. Marion arrived later in the afternoon, ran a few cursory tests and asked Calvin if he felt ready to leave. Calvin had no hesitation in saying he was ready to go and Dr. Marion obliged by signing the discharge form, she also wrote a letter so that Calvin could have access to the wheelchair service at the airport - he was going to need this. Dr. Marion also mentioned to Calvin that he was a lucky paediatric patient, who came and left in 2 days, she could not remember when last someone did that in her ward. With that said I gave the kind Doctor the Mandela notebook, at least she showed appreciation as opposed to uncomfortable awkwardness. Liz sent me a message that she was on her way and wanted to help me take Calvin to the apartment, we quickly readied ourselves by getting Calvin dressed and packed. Getting dressed proved to be a rather tricky affair. By the time Liz arrived we were ready to go and so we made our way slowly down the ward passage past all the sick children. Earlier I had noticed that there were a group of people with older kids in the cafeteria partaking in what I thought was a small Christmas party. At the end of the passage one of the ladies stood looking fixedly at Calvin, she had a younger girl next to her, holding what seemed to be a present. As we drew nearer she approached us and started speaking in French, but thankfully our friend Liz was on hand to help translate. As they spoke I noticed that they were wearing T-shirts with an image of a young bald boy by the name of Donovan. Eventually Liz turned to me and said that they had a gift for Calvin and that he reminded her of her late son Donovan who would have been more or less his age. It was a touching moment. I let the complete stranger enjoy the experience of connecting with someone representing something so close to her heart. Apparently one of Donovan's wishes was that the paediatric ward be treated yearly to a Christmas party complete with presents and cake. We said our goodbyes and as we headed out of the ward I could still feel her eyes on Calvin as she struggled to break the brief connection. In anticipation Liz headed out first to collect her car so that she could collect us at the entrance, we were moving rather slowly as these were Calvin's first proper steps after his procedure. As I got close to the curb I could vaguely see Liz's car coming towards us, but in that moment Calvin's leg buckled and he fell to the ground. As I helped Calvin up, my heightened anxiety ratcheted up a notch.

The short drive to the apartment allowed us some time to chat to Liz, while her kids Gabriela and David made their way on the Paris Metro to visit Calvin. As Calvin climbed out of the car his first wobbly foothold was on wet paving and even with my assistance went tumbling to the ground once again, raising more concern from Liz. Once in the apartment hallway his leg once more folded like a limp noodle and this time he crashed into a wall. I tried to assure Liz that Calvin would in time get better and that she not worry, but internally I was worried. Once inside we unpacked and with that Liz got a call to collect the kids at the station. As she was about to leave Calvin asked if he could go for the ride and so the three of us made our way to the metro station. It wasn't long when we spotted them running hand-in-hand towards the car, their happiness filled the car instantly into a jovial bubble. From there we returned back to the apartment from where Liz began to unpack 'half-her-kitchen' out of the boot of her car. She went all out with salad, quiche, condiments and gifts for everyone. I stood there in disbelief as Liz has a highly pressured job on top of being a busy mother and now here she was mothering us. I tried my best to protest but she would have none of it and to cap things off she was insistent that she drop us off at the airport the next day. I think once again I had little to offer Liz, other than our gratitude. In our little apartment we all chatted and I could see that Calvin was enjoying the attention.

Liz and the kids eventually left us as they still had a long way to get home and we decided that as Calvin wanted a French croissant one more time for breakfast that we take a short walk to the nearby bakery. The time was by then 7:30 in the evening and the roads were still busy with traffic. We decided that we would go 'nice and slow' as it was both dark and wet. As we neared the bakery Calvin's leg once again gave way but I was ready this time and hung on to him. However, he replied "dad it's not my leg, I've slipped on something". Looking down I saw the unmistakable pile of dog poop now properly smeared all over Calvin's shoe, not to mention the most awful stench that went with it. The funny part was that before we left for Paris Charlene had warned Calvin about Parisian streets being magnets for dog poop. So here we were on our last night in the dark stepping on the Godzilla of all dog turds. Luckily Calvin found a puddle of water outside the bakery and while I got the croissants he vainly swished his shoe in the puddle to get some of the offending goo off. Walking in mirth back to our apartment we had to walk over a pedestrian crossing and in France one does not dilly-dally doing so. As we were halfway with cars both sides waiting for us, Calvin's foot momentarily miss-stepped sending me in the opposite direction to counter the fall which thankfully never occurred, but I imagined it looked suspiciously like a drunken spill to the impatient motorists. This made us laugh even more. Inside our toasty room we dined on Liz's kind offerings and went to bed content, it was our best night's sleep after our hospital ordeal.

The Long Road Home

We woke up late the next morning and I asked Calvin to lie on his back and try to raise his legs, one at a time. From that simple exercise it was immediately evident that the left leg was affected, he was unable to raise it a centimetre. I decided that we needed to go back to see the doctor at the hospital about this issue. Back at the paediatric ward Dr. Marion made Calvin walk up and down the corridor to which he obliged without a hitch, making me believe that I was overreacting. However, she prescribed compression socks for the journey and suggested I rub his leg with Voltaren gel. In her opinion it was nothing more than inflammation as result of the cryoablation to the left side of the sacral bone. With that we headed back one more time to our apartment and by this time Calvin seemed more sure-footed as he walked. As agreed Liz collected us in the early afternoon and headed straight to the airport. As it was the weekend before Christmas one could see the exodus of Parisians to the countryside, pretty much what we 'Joburgers' do on any given holiday. As I did not want to inconvenience Liz too much I suggested we go early so that at least she could return home earlier to her family. In typical Portuguese style Liz had laid out in a plastic container on her back seat baguette rolls crammed with fillings. Liz ensured that if anything we would leave France well fed. Once at the airport we headed straight to the wheelchair assist lounge where Calvin from then onwards did not have to worry about walking. We eventually stood at the departures entrance and Calvin expressed his gratitude for everything Liz and her family had done for him. It was a touching moment one in which I and I think even Liz struggled to keep tears at bay. We said our goodbyes, now it was just me and Calvin heading to our departure gate. Departure gates are probably the first point where one almost feels at home and it was no different on this occasion. The unmistakeable sounds of Afrikaans and Zulu welcomed us home.

Being wheelchair bound has its advantages, you get preferential treatment and Calvin had earned this honour. As we entered the aircraft a flight attendant with a sense of humour spotted Caleb's light-sabre in my backpack and proceeded to hum the *Star Wars* anthem replete with *Darth Vader's* asthmatic heavy-breathing. As

I was supporting Calvin by his arm in case he toppled-over, the next flight attendant made her own judgement and sternly asked Calvin "can you see me sir?" Once again there was mirth in the air as we joked about the attendant assuming that Calvin must be 'blind'. On our flight back we sat next to a trainee doctor studying in France, her name was Letta and she came from Limpopo. She was so intrigued about Calvin's condition that she took notes and asked many medical questions. Anyway I was thankful for this angel as she ensured that Calvin was always moving around and not sitting in one position. I was so tired that I had little energy to manage Calvin on the flight, but Letta had it all covered. Soon we were touching down in Johannesburg and once disembarked I lost sight of Letta in the crowds of people, and I still wonder to this day if it was all just a dream. Calvin once again got the handy wheelchair service and in no time we sailed past everyone through immigration and out into the waiting area where my dad was waiting.

The Panic Continues

It was nice to be back home again, especially since it was Christmas Eve and we were both looking forward to seeing Charlene and Caleb. The weather was balmy and our bodies quickly readjusted to the heat. Once home Calvin was showered in lots of love and attention. We even squeezed a walk around the block and everyone was happy. Later that evening my parents came over for dinner while we recounted our story to them and then we went straight to bed to stretch out our sore bodies. The following day we left for Bethal to meet up with Charlene's parents for Christmas Day, and from there on Boxing Day we would leave for our favourite spot on the coast, Pumula. Our optimism in Calvin's condition prior to us confirming our spot at the coast never accounted for the eventuality of his actual condition. Up to the point when we arrived at Pumula everything seemed to be progressing well. We had hardly settled into our coastal retreat when it was agreed that we would all go to the gym - a very bad idea indeed. During the hour gym session Calvin did a heavy workout, he was trying to pack all the pent-up energy of the last week into one session. The overwhelming energy that was being displayed was impressive but nonetheless worrying. Later that evening Calvin was in deep trouble, the pain had heightened and the pain killers were doing little to ease his suffering. This plunged Charlene and I into a new panic as there was little we could do for him at that stage. Thankfully as morning materialised I headed straight to the local chemist to get a knee brace for the inflammation and more anti-inflammatory tablets and creams. I somehow believed that inflammation was his biggest problem, but this was only part of the issue. Walking around the beach resort was almost impossible for Calvin and he spent most of his time on a deck chair around the pool or lying on his bed. To make matters worse Charlene had tried to contact local doctors who put the fear of the worst eventuality, namely the potential for neurological damage. Their suggestion was that he get to a hospital as soon as possible so that he could be medically assessed, the other suggestion was that we also terminate our holiday. We chatted and both agreed that we were not enjoying our holiday under the circumstances, the only one having the time of his life was Caleb and when he heard of our plan he was not happy at all.

That evening Calvin was dosed up with medication and we settled down for the night only to be woken up in the early hours of the morning with his groaning. We decided our best option was to drive him to the nearest hospital 80kms away at Amanzimtoti. We rolled the passenger chair down and made him as comfortable as possible. As we left the hotel premises in the dark I contemplated the possibility of nerve damage, but I eventually focused on the task of driving in the dark. Once we reached the emergency entrance to the Kingsway hospital an attendant quickly organised a wheelchair for Calvin and pushed him into one of the consultation cubicles. A doctor soon arrived and I started to explain Calvin's treatment in France, but as I was talking I realised that my story sounded fantastical and that this doctor might not even make sense of my story. My fear was compounded when asked "was this a trial based treatment?" And my immediate response was "no, certainly not, as it was approved by our medical aid even though it is not available in South Africa". The doctor then changed his approach when he mentioned that there was a neurologist on call and that he was going to first consult with him. The doctor then left us alone while I sat there looking at Calvin who was grimacing in pain and I thought back of the time many years ago when Calvin was two years old he landed up in the exact same hospital with a bronchial infection. He was a mere baby then and now here he was almost an adult, but still not out the woods in terms of his health. A short while later the doctor came in and said that after chatting to the neurologist the plan of action was that he would first put Calvin on a Paracetamol drip, if he responded then the problem would more than likely be acute inflammation of the nerve root. However, if he did not respond then the issue may be of a more severe nature and in that case they would transport him by ambulance to the main hospital in Durban. The doctor with the help of a nurse connected Calvin up to a drip and it was not too long before I could see the relief in Calvin's face as he started to even flex his leg naturally. This point in the whole ordeal was probably my high point, I now knew for a fact that it wasn't nerve damage and that we could work on this issue with time. The doctor whom I doubted had carried out his task as a professional and I was very grateful for that. Our trip back was relaxed as Calvin slept soundly as I watched the sunrise over the Indian Ocean and I knew all was going to be well. By the time I had arrived back at Pumula Charlene had already checked us out under the protestations of Caleb, she had also managed to get hold of Liz who kindly assisted us once more by getting hold of the French doctors.

An Abrupt End And A New Beginning
We left Pumula shortly after breakfast and while I drove to the nearest chemist to collect the prescribed corticosteroids, Caleb negotiated himself a PlayStation console in lieu of his aborted

holiday. As we stood to pay for the medication Charlene's phone rang, it was Dr. Tselikas the doctor who assisted Dr. Deschamps and specialises in embolization. Once the call was over Charlene looked at me and said that this was a normal reaction and that we should not worry, but to put him on the corticosteroids as soon as possible. Dr. Tselikas was also going to email us an updated prescription if needed. Charlene was upset that the French doctors had not provisioned for this to happen which resulted in unnecessary anxiety. She tried in vain to get our room back at Pumula but it was already taken since it was just before New Year's Eve and reluctantly we headed back to Charlene's parents in Bethal, however during the trip back we eventually felt comforted by the realisation that all was heading in the right direction for Calvin.

Two weeks later Calvin finished his course of medication and was progressing well. It was time for him to also start school and as walking was a major issue we tried to provision as best we could for this problem. Luckily his school friends assisted Calvin in carrying his bag between classes and this helped. We also started Calvin with physiotherapy and approached our biokineticist friend Tirene once more to help Calvin with his rehabilitation. Tirene is a biokineticist for the university that I also work for and helped to rehabilitate Calvin after his previous operation in Germany. This time around the university had invested in a large indoor pool for hydrotherapy and as Calvin required support for his back, water was the best place to get things started.

The year progressed rather quickly and Calvin pushed on with his schoolwork and his rehabilitation - we could see small but almost daily improvements. As Charlene was on the matric farewell committee one of her tasks was to organise a 'spinathon' event to raise funds and both our boys helped on the day. Unfortunately I worked that day but I did see some of the footage and to my amazement, saw Calvin, despite his limited movement partaking in cycling and aerobics classes with his younger brother.

Actually it is also his younger brother Caleb that should get some credit in keeping Calvin perpetually on his toes. In our backyard one will find miniature goal boxes and daily the brothers take each other on, complete while trash-talking each other's abilities. Obviously Calvin muscles his brother off the ball, but now Caleb had him in his sights. So Caleb would surreptitiously entice his brother to a friendly match and promise that he would go gentle on him. However, knowing Calvin, even if he was crawling he would still compete. For weeks on end Calvin hobbled helplessly around Caleb, while shot after shot found his goal. When I asked Caleb what he thought of Calvin's ability he retorted "he is a cripple you know, but I tell you he is getting better!". By April Calvin was growing frustrated in his disability and begged us to return to 5-a-side soccer, we relented but asked that he inform his team members that he was not yet fully recovered and if anything did not feel right he should stop. It wasn't too long before the brain-muscle connection was reaffirmed and Calvin was on his way to a full recovery. In the same month he joined the school cross-country team and was now getting the upper hand on his sly little brother at backyard soccer.

Confirming Good News

The Easter holidays soon followed and two rather large events lay in wait for Calvin. The first was the all-important scan to verify the result of the treatment and the second was being the master of ceremonies for the matric farewell dance. First Calvin did an MRI scan and then off we went back to the Steve Biko Academic hospital in Pretoria for the PET scan. These events went by quickly and then we waited for our radiologist oncologist Dr. Lohlun to summon us for a consultation. A week went by until we were seated in front of her waiting for her findings. The result was way beyond what we had hoped for, in place of the tumours now resided plastic material that supported his spine, no tumour activity was evident even from the highly sensitive PET scan. It was evident that Dr. Lohlun was very happy with the results and so should we have also been, however over the years we had learned to rather err on the side of caution. We were happy but we still needed the confirmation from Dr. Deschamps which we had to wait for another week while the scan disks made their way to him. I eventually received the long awaited email and as per usual it was to the point, but music to our ears, it went as follows "I had a look at the scans and totally agree (with Dr. Lohlun), this is good news". I can only describe the feeling I felt from my own perspective as I'm sure Calvin and Charlene experienced it slightly differently, but it was a bittersweet moment. For the first time in many years Calvin was tumour free and we could move forward as a family out of the constant grip of fear and the unknown. But this is not a movie so there is no ending, just another beginning.

In the time after our fantastic news Calvin eventually delivered his speech at the matric farewell in front of all his peers, teachers and parents. He relished every moment of this opportunity and exuded a quiet confidence usually reserved for someone much older. He was also later awarded first team colours for cross-country, something I would have thought impossible at the beginning of the year. For Calvin being able to walk across the stage with a big smile to collect his award was an achievement in itself, never mind the cross-country. On top of all this he continued with his excellent scholastic record despite personal setbacks and continues to dream of the possibilities for his future.

Today Calvin is a second year university student studying law, he achieved 7 distinctions in matric and 5 in his first year at university. As I write the concluding passages to this book I see him out in the garden doing handstands, not bad for someone with a compromised back. Despite the new challenge of COVID-19 we all face today he is determined to enjoy life as he wills. Ultimately, there are many people who we will always be indebted to, some are medical professionals, some are friends and family, others were complete strangers who we may never meet again. Our happiness stands as a testament to their efforts and kind interventions.

Thank you!

My Closing Thoughts

As humans we sometimes think that our problems are infinitely bigger than the next person's problems. We wonder and ask ourselves "why me, what did I do to deserve this upon myself?" In reality everyone has some sort of 'cross-to-bear' and I think that I am pretty happy carrying the burdens that I have already. I would really hate to shoulder some of the problems that other people have. This I have understood is what makes us all human - we are not perfect even if we think we are. Many times the thought has occurred to me that we may live forever, almost as if in perpetual motion. But life is more than that and we are definitely here in the passing. As such life throws you both highs and lows and you have the choice to learn from those experiences. This is the process of acquiring wisdom and as such wise people are those who have grown as result of life's tumultuous rhythms. So if ever you are faced with a crisis step back and ask "what is it that I am going to learn from this experience?"

In our case I have asked the question many times over and the realisation is that we have all learned something from this journey. I could list all those lessons but I will spare you the obvious. However, the most profound lesson for us as a family has been the twin lessons of faith and love. In our tribulation we unashamedly turned to our faith. Those dark cold winter nights when Charlene and I wandered around the house sobbing, it was in our personal faith that we sought refuge. We pleaded, we asked, we cried. It was a very basic process and it embodied our faith more than any religious practice. In fact I'm the first to admit that my Christian upbringing has been tempered by logical enquiry and as such I tend to be a sceptic – an agnostic if you wish. Charlene on the other hand has always been the devout Christian. But despite the differences in belief system we knew that miracles could not happen without us exerting energy to find them.

Love was the other big lesson we had to learn. We realised that without our friends and family we would be lost. It is because of our friends love for our family that we were able to focus with faith in healing Calvin. Love was manifested in a variety of ways to us and these included prayer, gifts, words of affirmation and practical support. So many of you prayed for us, from Calvin's school, Charlene's mom, Charlene's friends, Kirsten, Dennis, Jayne, Celeste, Henriette, Liesl and many more, my mom and sisters, the list is ongoing. Our daily food gifts sustained us and came in handy when our house had numerous impromptu visitors. The gift bearers that kept us going included, Isabel and Amy, Meryl, Sonnel, Prina, Priel and their mom, Jenny and Amanda. Many of you reflected your love through words of affirmation in particular Calvin's friends Amy, Julio, Alex, Florian and Ehren, Malcolm and Wanita, Danie and Gerda, Ines and Gerard, and Tanja's mom Hermien. Without practical support it would have been difficult to have achieved what we did in such a short time and without doubt Joerg and Tanja's contribution was immense, others included Henriette, Lora, Charlene's parents who looked after Caleb (sadly her dad passed away last year) and my father Eugenio who kept things at home ticking effortlessly. We also cannot forget our Parisian friends Liz, Michael and kids – we would truly be alone without your support in a foreign city.

Love was also showered upon us by complete strangers. Henriette's mom Chrissie was at the forefront of her prayer group in the UK and they did hard work on their knees on our behalf. People with differing beliefs supported us, be they Christian, Hindu, Muslim or Atheist, love was exposed. The nurses and doctors that we met in South Africa, Germany and France showed their love in their caring for Calvin. As such we have grown new friendships, amazing people that we could have never have met if it were not for our personal struggle. To all these people we are privileged to count on you as friends. Such is life.

EPILOGUE

As I near my seventeenth birthday I have realised that I have received deep knowledge and wisdom that transcends beyond my years which have ultimately made me into the person I am today. This wisdom stems from my countless experiences with hardship. If I hadn't crossed paths with these obstinate hardships I would not have the 'strong-resilient' characteristics that form the foundation of my current identity. These experiences that I have faced have allowed me to view the world as a whole with both its empowering and debilitating facets. I have gained significant inner strength which has given me a higher degree of patience and courage in the face of adversity. Sometimes I think this may have been the best thing that has ever happened to me. It has opened my eyes to who I really am and what I was meant to accomplish. I have successfully been able to turn a tragedy into a window of opportunity. I am Calvin dos Santos and this is my story.

I was thirteen when I was told I had a rare adrenal tumour sitting wedged between my vital organs. This tumour had grown as result of a genetic predisposition. My condition needed immediate attention due to the immense amount of adrenaline being 'pumped' into my system which had me on the verge of cardiac arrest. Doctors explained that removing the tumour would involve a risky procedure of taking out internal organs in hope of reaching the enlarged growth. "This can't be happening to me" is what I remember thinking. I was fit, I was healthy and I thought I was invincible. The prospect of the operation being successful was very slim and death seemed imminent. Being as young as I was, I felt a sinking dread, a panic that seemed to rise and fall with each struggled breath. All my hope was drained out of me and I seemingly felt the dagger of dread turning in my stomach, inflicting a pain that was incomprehensible. I lost all my direction and started to accept the worst outcome. When you find yourself so close to death's hands you start to ascertain who you really are.

My parents continued to seek an approach that adeptly removed my growth and that allowed me to live a so-called "normal" life. By reading an innumerable amount of medical papers and spending hours on the phone with various medical institutions planted around the world; a positive ray of light materialised. It was through their ceaseless determination that they were able to find a team of experts in Germany who advocated a minimally invasive procedure. I was flown to Germany within a few weeks and propelled on the road to self-discovery. Soon I was wheeled into the operating room donning my white robe. I can't remember very much but I do remember the cold feeling of alcohol being rubbed on my arm, a sharp prick and then the white, milky liquid languidly inching its way through my veins. Suddenly a drowsy feeling overcame me and my eyelids struggled to hold themselves open. Before I completely passed out I remember seeing a path to a better life laid out in front of me. No one would have blamed me if I wallowed in self-pity. But I saw a way out and grabbed it. I started to realise that despite everything I would have gone through, I was still determined to be the same person I was. I was determined to have my humour and life back again. This was when I had unearthed my true identity - I was a fighter.

I woke up with a reverberating pain that pulsed through me, each wave more powerful and painful than the last. A throbbing pain seemed to be accumulating near my lower back. I tried to sit up but I felt as if a heavy force kept me planted on the mattress. Screaming was a futile effort as my voice was hoarse. My lips had garnered lumps of dried saliva which had been as result of the constant insert and exit of pipes supplying oxygen or draining bodily fluids. My eyes seemed to be frozen open and I tried to take in all my surroundings. Long wires of pipes were coiled around me from the balls of my fists and spanning into my inner nostrils. Every moment or so, a new face appeared above me, muttering something foreign to the person beside them with a clipboard and adjusting the monitors that ominously blinked with my frayed heartbeat. Moments seemed blurry and sometimes I couldn't tell if I had drifted into an unconscious state. The doctors later told me that the procedure had spanned over eleven hours and I was verging on the state of a heart attack due to the excessive stress hormones that the tumour was producing even as it was being taken apart.

I can still remember the cold dread of those days being confined to a hospital bed. During these arduous periods, I gained insightful knowledge. I started to discover the small things which I had always taken for granted. I started to acknowledge and appreciate life more. Around me, other patients were dying in those white-walled facilities. Balding children with hardened faces were connected to IV drips that oozed a white liquid into their veins as they ambled through the hallways with a sombre frailty. I had so much to be thankful for and a refusal to give up a fight makes me the person I am today.

After I had conquered life's daily challenges that set me apart from other people, I relished new ones. In Victor Frankl's book Man's search for meaning, Frankl describes the life in a Nazi concentration camp and how the inmates were able to withstand torture and tough conditions because they were able to cope by somehow finding meaning in tragedy. Frankl goes on to explain that "Everything can be taken from a man, but for one thing, the last of the human freedoms - to choose one's attitude in any given set of circumstances, to choose one's own way."

You don't need a near death experience to find your own identity or start again. I wish everyone could get on that page. Although I am fighting a constant battle with illness, I am always trying to do what others may be taking for granted. I am living my life with limitless possibilities and enduring life's constant battles thrown my way. Even though I am fully aware that genetics are against me, I also know that I have one thing that stands in its way. My refusal to give up hope and the fighter that lives in me. My identity.

"The fighter that lives in me" piece written by Calvin for school - March 2017.

AFTERWORD

A parent's love is one of the strongest and most uncompromising kinds of love you will ever come across, and it is only when the wellbeing of a child is threatened that you realise the determination that a parent has. But for me the determination came from a belief in the power of prayer supported by faith. How absolutely devastated Victor and I were to hear Calvin's diagnosis. It was a serious dose of reality! The sense that you have to do all you can for Calvin to get better, but how at the same time much is left out of your hands. I can only say that my faith kept me strong throughout the whole ordeal. I lit a candle every day with an inscription that read "Faith does not make things easy, but it does make it possible". These words helped to keep me focused on the arduous task ahead.

Our family and friends supported us throughout our journey, helping us to cope daily. Calvin's school, De la Salle Holy Cross were so supportive and we will be forever grateful for their prayers throughout our journey. Calvin's illness was transformed from a physical to a spiritual quest and became a process which united our minds, hearts and souls. The way in which doors were opened for angels in the walking to be sent our way reassured in us that Calvin's healing was a miracle.

Charlene dos Santos - July 2013

HOW TO BEAT CANCER
IN 7 BASIC STEPS

The list to follow is similar to what we followed and we still apply some of the basics to Calvin's yearly preventative screening. Also to consider is the fact that before any of these steps can take place there should be obvious health signs that may be of concern to you. Parents and in particular mothers are well equipped to detect abnormal signs evident in their children. Our experience is also particular to adrenal tumours and resultant metastatic bone cancer, so screening and treatment options can vary vastly. However, the stepped approach is a good start for anyone wanting medical answers with a viable solution.

Step 1 – Initial Screening
Your first option here is to see your family doctor and describe the symptoms that are observable. Your doctor at this stage will run baseline tests and possibly order blood tests. This can be a problematic stage as in our experience first line doctors were not equipped to consider further health issues when their baseline tests showed good health. If there is a genetic link that may be known at the time then taking this evidence to your doctor will save much time and frustration in achieving a correct diagnosis. The experience with my sister in the UK demonstrated how the use of family medical evidence to correlate with existing symptoms facilitated the diagnosis.

Step 2 – Diagnosis
You may get an initial diagnosis from your family doctor and

hopefully a referral to a specialist physician. If you are not completely satisfied go back to step 1 and get a second opinion.

Step 3 – Further screening by specialist physician

At this stage once the diagnosis is confirmed and you are in the hands of a specialist physician like a paediatric endocrinologist screening options will be vast and tailored to the particular type of cancer. Options for screening include targeted blood tests to look at various stress hormone levels, 24-hour urine tests, 24-hour blood pressure tests, HBA1C long-term blood glucose level, MRI scan, CT scan, PET-CT scan and possibly a nuclear medicine scan (MIBG). These are all critical in compiling a composite 'image' of the extent of the cancer and key to the success of step 4.

Step 4 – Treatment options and planning

This stage also presents many options depending on the type of cancer diagnosed, the health of the patient and the extent of the disease. You also need to be at your sharpest here as you and your loved ones will have the final say as to what the best approach will be for the best outcome. Some treatments will result in lifetime detriments so these need to be weighed up carefully if indeed critical. Options for treatment include surgery (invasive or non-invasive), chemotherapy, radiation therapy, nuclear medicine (MIBG), ablation therapy, embolization and specific drug protocols. Treatments can be selected only if your type of cancer responds well, your physician will guide you extensively on these, but you will also have the power to do your own research. A word of advice here is to avoid trial based treatments as these are experimental, so opt for treatments that are clinically proven and have much research literature in support of positive outcomes. Once options have been assessed it will be inevitable that the medical centres offering these treatments will already be chosen. Do not limit your options, look at what is available globally. Our experience bears testament to this approach. You will find that local medical centres will offer treatments like chemotherapy, but other treatments may be out of their specialisation realm.

Step 5 – Treatment

Once your centre of excellence and medical team has been chosen and an appropriate date has been set for treatment, you and the rest of the family must prepare for any eventualities. These may include extended stays in hospital, treatment option changes due to complications, but this list can be extensive. I am hoping for best outcomes so once you're in the system usually it's just a progression of events. Your planning and family support will pay dividends at this stage. You and your family will have limited expertise at this stage, leave it up to the professionals. Your expertise will be love, humility, understanding and support. You will also need to be well prepared for the next stage as you are not 'out-of-the woods' yet.

Step 6 – Recovery

The first level to this stage if surgery was performed is transitioning through ICU. Your input here is usually limited as there are strict rules to entry, but you may get permission in paediatric cases. Once your physician is happy with the results at ICU a move to the hospital ward is the next step. In the normal ward the nurses and other medical attendants will support the recovery process, and when possible mobilisation will be absolutely crucial for healing. On the psychological side the support and care from loved ones goes without question and keeping an active mind busy with activities will make time pass-by quicker.

If receiving radiation, chemo or nuclear therapy you will more than likely experience recovery at home. In my opinion this will be more comfortable and offer more options in terms of family support. You could also use the opportunity to incorporate alternative methods that support a healthy recovery, these could include supplementation, better food options, meditation and exercise.

Step 7 – Preventative screening

Congratulations, remission or stable-disease is confirmed and life goes back to normal...but not so fast. Once a cancer has been diagnosed and treated successfully your work does not end here. Healthy living habits coupled with a preventative screening protocol managed by your chosen physician will be paramount to living a normal life. Oncology centres are good in this regard, but physicians like endocrinologists can also be helpful. The main criteria here is that there is mutual trust and respect established and that you are able to access the doctor easily should any concern arise.

CENTRES OF MEDICAL EXCELLENCE

From our experience these are your 'go-to' centres of excellence. Some have an excellent reputation when it comes to treating 'rare' types of cancer. The European centres from our varied experiences are world leaders in cutting-edge medical technologies. If you would like to contact me regarding our experience with a particular centre I would only be too happy to oblige.

Please email me on: **how2beatcancerbook@gmail.com**

Germany:
Freiburg Academic Clinic - https://www.uniklinik-freiburg.de/de.html
Essen-Mitte Clinic - https://kem-med.com/

France:
Gustav Roussy Cancer Campus Paris - https://www.gustaveroussy.fr/
Strasbourg University Hospital - http://www.chru-strasbourg.fr/

South Africa:
Donald Gordon Mediclinic - https://www.mediclinic.co.za/en/wits-donald-gordon-medical-centre/home.html
Red Cross Childrens Hospital - http://www.paediatrics.uct.ac.za/scah/clinicalservices/medical/oncology

United Kingdom:

Royal Free Hospital London - https://www.royalfree.nhs.uk/

United States:
Children's Hospital of Philadelphia - https://www.chop.edu/

THANK YOU

First of all, thank you for purchasing my book *How to beat cancer*. I know you could have picked any number of books to read, but you picked this book and for that I am extremely grateful.

I hope that it adds inspiration and hope to your everyday life. If so, it would be really nice if you could share this book with your friends and family by posting the link to Facebook and Twitter.

If you enjoyed this book and found some benefit in reading it, I'd like to hear from you and hope that you could take some time to post a review on Amazon. Your feedback and support will help me as an author to greatly improve my writing craft for future projects and make this book even better.

I once again thank you humbly for your support and wish you all the best for the future. Hope to hear from you when my next book is released!

Victor dos Santos - July 2020